The Phy... Challenge

M000239801

Book I:
A Chance for Redemption:
Contributions of Men Behind Bars

Book II:
Discovery is Our Business

Richard L. DeGowin

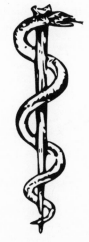

Ice Cube Press, LLC
North Liberty, Iowa, USA

The Physician's Challenge:
A Chance for Redemption—Contributions of Men Behind Bars
& Discovery is Our Business

Copyright ©2021 Richard L. DeGowin, MD
First Edition
Isbn 9781948509244
Library of Congress Control Number: 2021935639

Ice Cube Press, LLC (Est. 1991)
1180 Hauer Drive
North Liberty, Iowa 52317 USA
www.icecubepress.com | steve@icecubepress.com

All rights reserved.

No portion of this book may be reproduced in any way
without permission, except for brief quotations for review, or
educational work, in which case the publisher shall be provided
copies. The views expressed in *The Physician's Challenge* are
solely those of the author, not the Ice Cube Press, LLC.

The paper used in this publication meets the minimum requirements of the American National Standard
for Information Sciences—Permanence of Paper for
Printed Library Materials, ANSI Z39.48-1992.

Manufactured in USA using recycled paper.

Note on cover image: The Staff of Aesculapius (the Greek god
of medicine), is a serpent entwined around it. It is the symbol of
medicine.

The Physician's challenge is the curing of disease, educating people in the laws of health, and preventing the spread of plagues and pestilences.
—Sir William Osler

Dedicated
to the men who volunteered for studies
and served on the staff of the
Malaria Project,

and

to the doctors whose stories I tell with
admiration and affection.

Author's Note

For a nurse to inject you with a safe and effective vaccine protective against infection of COVID19 virus, the developer of the vaccine undertook an experiment—required by law—in which thousands of persons at risk of contracting the viral illness, received injections of the vaccine or injections of a placebo (no active substance). The number of persons who were protected and the number of those who tested positive for the virus were compared and recorded. This is *human experimentation*—called *clinical trials*—to appease those who might be put off by the former phrase.

Contents—Book I: A Chance for Redemption

Dedication

Preface.. 11

Introduction.. 19

Part I. Fort Sam Houston (1963 July 5-23) 25

Billets, Classes, & Courtesy............................. 26

Doctors Under Fire....................................... 38

Graduation & Leave....................................... 47

Part II. Stateville (1963-1964)........................... 50

Prologue.. 50

Plainfield, Illinois...................................... 54

The Malaria Project....................................... 62

The Prison Community...................................... 75

Malaria and its Vector.................................... 82

The Volunteers.. 89

Professor Alf S. Alving, MD, Director..................... 95

Tuesdays.. 98

Our Fallen Chief.. 103

Part III. Stateville (1964-1965)......................... 110

Prologue.. 110

Eureka!... 111

Bioethics... 123

Recapitulation.. 133

Civil Rights.. 139

Walter Reed Army Institute of Research.................... 142

The Decision.. 146

Part IV. The Job (1965).................................. 150

Interviews.. 150

The University of Chicago................................. 155

Epilogue.. 158

Appendix One 162

Appendix Two 167

Bibliography... 167

Book Two:

Discovery is Our Business 177

ILLINOIS STATE PENITENTIARY
JOLIET-STATEVILLE BRANCH
JOLIET, ILLINOIS

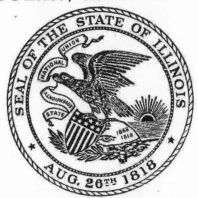

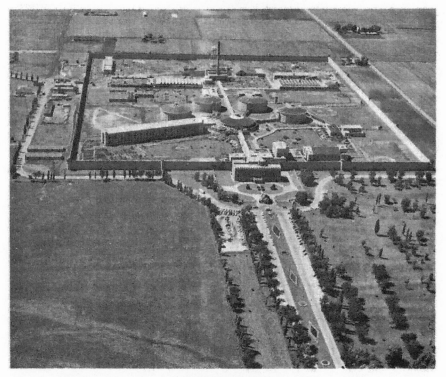

STATEVILLE PENITENTIARY

Stateville Penitentiary Joliet, Illinois; 1960's

Preface

On 5 February 1958, in his fifth appearance before the Parole Board, Nathan Leopold said, in part, "...All I want in this life is a chance to prove to you and the people of Illinois, what I know in my own heart to be true, that I can and will become a decent, self-respecting and law-abiding citizen, to have a chance to find redemption for myself by service to others. It is for that chance that I humbly beg."*

In petitioning for his release from Stateville Penitentiary, his lawyer, Elmer Gertz, pointed out that since his incarceration, Nathan Leopold had served mankind during his life sentence plus 99 years for the kidnapping and brutal murder of Bobby Franks. He had developed a school for inmates, he had worked as an x-ray technician and as a psychiatric nurse in the prison hospital, and he had volunteered to take malaria during research studies on the Malaria Project.

Nathan Leopold was 19 years old when he entered prison. After serving 33 years, he was released from Stateville Penitentiary on parole, 13 March 1958. He accepted a job as a medical assistant in the mission hospital of the Church of the Brethren in Castaner, a village high in the mountains of Puerto Rico, far away from the reporters who, on his release from prison, hounded his every step in Illinois.

On a cold day in February, a letter arrived in my mailbox addressed to the "Officer-in-Charge, Malaria Project, Illinois State Penitentiary, Box 1112, Joliet, Illinois." The letter, signed by Nathan Leopold, dated

---

* Gertz, Elmer: *A Handful of Clients*, Follett, Chicago, 1965, p. 100; quoted in, Baatz, Simon: *For the Thrill of It, Leopold, Loeb, and the Murder That Shocked Chicago*, Harper Collins, New York, 2008, p. 442.

8 February 1965, seven years after his discharge from Stateville, he wrote he was employed as a Research Assistant in the Social Science Program, Office of Scientific Investigation, Department of Health, Commonwealth of Puerto Rico. (See facing page.)

Intending to undertake drug-testing experiments using prisoners in the local penitentiary as volunteer subjects, similar to studies on the Malaria Project at Stateville, he requested a copy of the "release," like the one he had signed when he volunteered to take malaria there in the spring of 1945. The document we used described the benefits to society and the risks to the volunteer, governing our conduct of studies on human beings, dictated by the rules of the Nuremberg Code and the Declaration of Helsinki.

The Nuremberg Code for the conduct of research on human subjects, developed from the trials of Nazi war criminals after World War II, was read to inmates volunteering to take malaria, and it was included in the document each volunteer signed in duplicate before witnesses, who then signed it in turn.

The letter I held then told me Nathan Leopold was seeking "to find redemption" for the crime he committed that resulted in his incarceration. As I read his letter, I reflected upon the associations I had with this writer whom I had never met.

At the moment I received the letter, I stood in the Conference Room of the Malaria Project on the third floor of Stateville's prison hospital where Leopold had signed on to take malaria. As a medical student at The University of Chicago, I had lived only blocks from the Hyde Park Neighborhood where Leopold and Loeb had grown up and gone to school. Richard Loeb, who masterminded the murder of Bobby Franks in 1924, had transferred from The University of Chicago to The University of Michigan in Ann Arbor for his last two

COMMONWEALTH OF PUERTO RICO
DEPARTMENT OF HEALTH
SAN JUAN, PUERTO RICO

Social Science Program
Office of Scientific Investigation

February 8, 1965

The Officer-in-Charge
Malaria Project
Illinois State Penitentiary
Box 1112
Joliet, Illinois

Dear Sir:

      I am at present employed as Research Associate in the Social Science Program, Office of Scientific Investigation, Department of Health, Commonwealth of Puerto Rico.

      We intend, in the very near future, to perform some drug-testing experiments using prisoners of the local penitentiary as volunteer subjects. These experiments will, in many ways, be similar to the experiments carried on in Stateville on the therapy of malaria.

      It would be most helpful to our department if you could send me a copy of the release used by the Malaria Project and signed by the individual inmate volunteer.

      Thanking you in advance for your kindness in this matter,

Sincerely yours,

Nathan F. Leopold
Research Associate

NFL:mem

Letter from Nathan Leopold requesting document of informed consent.

years of college. He had lived at the ZBT Jewish Fraternity, where, 30 years later, my roommate at Michigan and I attended a party one evening. Loeb graduated from the College of Literature, Science and the Arts of The University of Michigan in the spring of 1923, in the same class as my mother and father, and returned to Chicago for graduate studies.

Leopold told members of the Parole Board in 1958 he sought a chance to find redemption by *leaving* Stateville. In an odd way of thinking about it, perhaps I looked for some sort of redemption by *entering* Stateville to work in 1963. My path to Stateville began at age 18½, about the same age Leopold was incarcerated.

PAYBACK TIME

Every year since 1952, the year I turned 18 and registered for the Selective Service, I had received a letter from Local Board 13-52, in Iowa City, Iowa, asking me to divulge my plans for education. While my peers served in Korea and elsewhere during the Cold War, other students like me had been granted deferment from active duty in the Army to complete our education, which I alleged would make my service more valuable to the Army and my country. It was. Well, now, after ten years of deferment, it was payback time.

As a Fellow doing physiological research related to erythropoiesis in Dr. Clifford Gurney's laboratory at The University of Chicago, there was little opportunity for me to learn the biochemistry of the red blood cell. Cliff suggested I could remedy that deficiency by joining Dr. Alf S. Alving, Director of the University of Chicago-Army Medical Research Project, and fulfill my active duty service obligation simultaneously.

Dr. Alving's group had documented the curative effects of the antimalarial drug, Primaquine. In the course of their studies on its toxicity, a member of the group, Dr. Paul Carson, discovered an erythrocyte enzymopathy, glucose-6-phosphate dehydrogenase deficiency, predisposing the red blood cells of certain persons to destruction when they ingested the drug. As a medical student, resident, and fellow, at The University of Chicago, I shared with my peers the excitement and pride in the Alving group's international recognition for these important discoveries.

The Visit

Dr. Alving offered me the opportunity to serve as a medical officer on the Army Medical Research Project of The University of Chicago, starting 1 July 1963. I would replace Captain George Brewer, MD, whose discharge from active duty was scheduled then. Before making my decision to accept Dr. Alving's offer, I was invited to visit the Malaria Project and meet and discuss the service with the medical officers, Dr. Robin D. Powell and Dr. George Brewer.

In addition to being impressed during my visit with the Project, its staff and its facilities, two things come to mind. Whereas current work on the Project concentrated on drug toxicity studies of red blood cell biochemistry, Robin mentioned recent reports of infections by drug-resistant malaria in several medical officers assigned to stations in Southeast Asia. He said they might require investigation on the Project.

The other thing I noted later at lunch in the Officers' Dining Room was the palpable sense of relief and good feelings in the guards and administrators dining at nearby tables. They had learned Governor Otto J. Kerner had just commuted the sentence of an inmate scheduled to be electrocuted at Stateville that morning.

After returning to our apartment to discuss our future with Karen, I wrote the following letter:

9237 South Laflin St.

Chicago 20, Illinois

August 22, 1962 (Wed.)

Dear Robin D. Powell, MD,

I appreciated your showing me the "Stateville Post-graduate School of Medicine" yesterday. The careful work which you have done with G-3-PD (Glyceraldehyde-3-Phosphate Dehydrogenase) is particularly interesting.

This afternoon I accepted Dr. Alving's offer, and I will plan to enter the Army July 1, 1963 for assignment to Stateville until July 1, 1965.

I am grateful to both George and you for speaking frankly with me and for your advice. I will look forward to seeing you when you come to Chicago and to working with you next year.

Sincerely,

Dick

Richard L. DeGowin, MD

CAPTAIN'S COMMISSION

In 1962, with Dr. Alving's help, I volunteered for the Doctor's Draft and applied for a commission as Captain, U.S. Army Medical Corps, assignment to Walter Reed Army Institute of Research, with duty station in Joliet, Illinois. At that time, the government drafted doctors to active service in the Army until age 36 years. The course of my application took me to U.S. Fifth Army Headquarters at 1660 East Hyde Park Boulevard in an old but grand structure near The University of Chicago Campus within a block or so of beautiful Lake

Michigan. Little did I realize then, as I walked through the halls of this impressive building, that heroes of the Civil War, the Indian Wars and Spanish American Wars had preceded me: General Philip H. (Little Phil) Sheridan, General Nelson A. Miles, and probably, General John J. (Black Jack) Pershing. General Pershing lived in our neighborhood at 337 East 53rd Street after his service in Zamboanga, the Philippines.

Ordered to the Army Induction Center at 615 N. Van Buren Street in Chicago on Tuesday, 20 November 1962, for a physical examination and fingerprinting, I sat in a classroom with a group of young men 8-10 years my junior, filling out forms. At age 28, I felt old.

The seasoned Master Sergeant anticipated our questions about various items on the numbered lines of the forms and said, "In the section on brothers and sisters, start by listing the eldest first. If you've got more than five, forget the rest. In the section asking you to list the names of your children, start with the eldest. If you've got more than five, forget 'em."

As the only physician in our group, I was honored by my professional brother, a uniformed medical officer, who examined me for inguinal hernia *first*, before continuing his examinations of the rest of us, standing in line with our pants down. Completing the physical examination, now dressed, I was addressed by a friendly young Captain in the Medical Corps seated at a desk.

He said, "I see you are a medical resident at The University of Chicago Hospital, the thinking man's hospital. I'm from Cook County Hospital, the doing man's hospital."

"Have you ever flunked a doctor?" I asked.

"One," he replied. "He was obese with diabetes, high blood pressure, and a bleeding duodenal ulcer."

This case must have been an exception, because Army policy was, "If you are healthy enough to practice medicine as a civilian, you are healthy enough to practice in the Army."

Introduction

I feel compelled to tell this story, because what I experienced can never happen again, and it recalls to my mind a noble effort of men who worked together to complete an important mission.

"First, Do No Harm," guides physicians in their care of patients, but while on active duty in the army, I joined medical officers who administered a disease to volunteer prison inmates in order to find a cure for malaria. How did all this come about, and how did I reconcile my oath as a doctor with my commitment to this mission? We were aware that Nazi doctors, convicted of war crimes, had been hung for conducting experiments on prisoners who did *not* volunteer for studies in Germany during World War II. Before the war, malaria had been given to other subjects in Europe, most of whom had not given their consent to receive the disease.

Julius Wagner-Jauregg, an Austrian psychiatrist, received the 1927 Nobel Prize in Medicine. He showed that the immune response associated with the high fevers of malaria—a disease he gave to his young male patients suffering from the insanity of advanced (general paresis) syphilis—cured 30% of them, enabling them to return to a productive family life instead of dying within two years of the onset of dementia from this prevalent aggressive venereal disease. As a result, malaria therapy for the insanity of advanced syphilis was adopted by physicians at mental institutions throughout the world, including Manteno State Hospital in Illinois.

Malaria killed more than a million persons each year, especially non-immune children in Africa and in other tropical areas throughout the world. Thus, there was a pressing need to discover drugs capable of preventing and curing the disease. Scientists had successfully propagated mammalian cells in tissue culture, but they were unable to keep malarial parasites alive for drug studies *in vitro*. Experiments with strains of malaria naturally infecting chickens, ducks, and mice, failed to predict efficacy and toxicity of new drugs administered to patients with malaria. It became clear to doctors that to have any value, studies had to be carried out in human beings.

Induced malaria infections were controlled with a standard antimalarial drug in syphilitic patients receiving malarial therapy to cure their insanity. So, physician investigators administered, new, potentially effective antimalarial drugs to syphilitic patients receiving malaria therapy in hopes that the test results would prove applicable to patients who had contracted the disease from the bites of infected mosquitoes. But when these patient subjects received malaria, they were ill with syphilis and other diseases, some dying of their affliction, obscuring the results as to whether a potential antimalarial drug was effective or toxic.

World War II

During World War II, malaria devastated U.S. Marines and U.S. Army troops on Guadalcanal in the Pacific Theater of Operations, putting hundreds of our men in hospital with malaria instead of on the frontline fighting the Japanese.

Early in the war, Japanese captured the cinchona plantations in Java, denying the Americans and British the antimalarial quinine. Atabrine, a 9-aminoacridine dye, produced by the I.G. Farbenindustrie in Germany, and Winthrop in the United States, was a suppressive, non-curative antimalarial drug administered to our troops if they could be induced to accept its side-effects—nausea, vomiting, hallucinations, yellowing of skin, and a rumor it caused impotence. Doctors found that lower doses prevented malaria and reduced side-effects except for the yellow skin. The saying was, "It's better to be yellow than dead."

So, in 1944, Alf Sven Alving, MD, an expert on kidney disease, recently recruited to the medical faculty of The University of Chicago from The Rockefeller Institute, where he had worked with the famous Dr. Donald Van Slyke, was tasked by the U.S. Army to establish the Malaria Project at Stateville Penitentiary, Joliet, Illinois.

With the voluntary participation of prison inmates in studies of antimalarial drugs, and with the work of medical officers and nurses on the University of Chicago-Army Medical Research Project in Stateville, the group confirmed the curative and preventive effects of Primaquine, an 8-aminoquinoline. In addition, they discovered that its side-effect, Primaquine-sensitive hemolysis, which occurred in 10% of black men taking the drug, was caused by a sex-linked genetic defect in red blood cell metabolism, glucose-6-phosphate dehydrogenase (G-6-PD) deficiency. This research on the antimalarial drug studies with volunteer inmates received widespread publicity in the national and Chicago press, in reports printed in American medical journals, and in World Health Organization (WHO) publications.

Vietnam

When I considered joining the research group at Stateville in 1962, the focus of its investigations was on the effects of drugs and their toxicity on the metabolism of the red blood cell—basic research with important clinical application.

By the time I joined the group in July 1963, the early reports of widespread multidrug resistant malaria infecting soldiers and civilians in Vietnam, Malaya, in other parts of Southeast Asia, and even in Brazil, had been confirmed and documented.

This represented not only a major global health challenge, but it was of great concern to officers in the U.S. Army Medical Corps, because President John F. Kennedy had expanded the number of military personnel deployed in Vietnam from 385 Americans, ordered there by President Eisenhower in the 1950's who served in MACV (Military Advisory Command Vietnam), to 17,000 troops by 1963. It soon became apparent that the focus of research at the Army Medical Research Project of The University of Chicago would shift to emphasize a search for drugs to prevent and cure multidrug resistant malaria.

RESEARCH WITH HUMAN SUBJECTS

Finding an effective treatment for this mutated parasite was of importance, not only to the military, but a new drug could save thousands of the lives of persons living in the tropics where malaria was endemic. Studies of malaria in human subjects had been undertaken safely for 20 years on the Malaria Project in Stateville's tightly controlled prison hospital. The studies were not carried out in secrecy, but in fact received widespread publicity in the lay press, the radio, and in scientific journals: *Life Magazine*, *WGN* (Chicago), American and World Health Organization medical journals. President Harry S. Truman had awarded Dr. Alving The Presidential Certificate of Merit for his work on malaria at Stateville. The Malaria Project depended upon the support of the Surgeon General of the U.S. Army, The University of Chicago, and the Illinois Bureau of Prisons.

Stateville's Prison Administration appreciated that more than 95% of the inmates whose lives they were temporarily caring for would eventually return to society. To that end, inmates enrolled for vocational training, attended school to earn a high school diploma (GED), and even to acquire credits for up to 3 years of college courses, or they worked in the prison industries, learning a work ethic and skills they could market for employment in the outside world.

No one coerced inmates to participate in the studies of the Malaria Project. Invariably, when announcements of malaria studies were posted on bulletin boards, more than twice as many inmates volunteered than could be accepted. Those who took malaria could not donate blood to the blood banks from The University of Chicago and Northwestern University Hospitals, which collected blood from inmates before the time that the prevalence of hepatitis-B precluded participation. Blood donors received a modest stipend to use in the Prison Commissary, unavailable to volunteers who took malaria. On completion of a malaria study, a letter commending his service to mankind was placed in the inmate's file for review by the Parole Board. It was not a, "Get out of jail free card." Members of the Parole Board had read many of the letters written for the 4,000 inmates who had volunteered to participate in studies on malaria since their inception in 1944.

When I asked one of our inmate clerks, "Why would an inmate volunteer to take malaria?" He said, "Some of them have brothers in the army, some seek redemption for their sins through service to mankind, but would rarely admit it, and some do it, because the 'man-on-the-street' would be afraid to do it, a macho thing. Others see it as a change in their routine life—hospitalized, socializing with other volunteers, eating good food, and visited several times daily by doctors and nurses concerned for their care and comfort. Most consider their ability to volunteer a right. Their rights are assured by a number of advocates—their lawyers, inmate support groups, and chaplains of every religious persuasion assigned to Stateville."

During the two years I served on active duty on the Army Medical Research Project of The University of Chicago, and during the 54 years since then, I have come to realize that I worked with a team of colleagues and volunteer inmates who confronted an important problem, and together found a solution that prevented suffering and benefited society.

Part I. Fort Sam Houston
(5-23 July 1963)

Orders by the Commander of Headquarters Fifth United States Army at 1660 East Hyde Park Boulevard, Chicago, Illinois, dated 17 April 1963, stated in part:

> *Subject: Active Duty*
> *To: Captain Richard L. DeGowin, MC, USAR*
> DeGowin, Richard L.,----5229, Captain MC, USAR, MOSC-3139 Ready Reserve
> *TDY enroute to: Medical Field Service School (3410),*
> *Brooke Army Medical Center,*
> *Fort Sam Houston, Texas*
> *Reporting date (TDY): Not earlier than 3JUL63 and not later than 5JUL63*
> *Course: AMEDS Orientation Course 8-A-C20A*

After graduating from high school, I wrote to the Johnson County Selective Service Board every year for the next ten years requesting deferment from the military draft to complete my formal education. "The more professional education you have, the better you will be able to serve your country," Bob Hardin, (WWII Veteran and Dean, College of Medicine, The University of Iowa) told me. Now, at the advanced age of 29 years, it was payback time. My Captain's Commission was dated 8 April 1963.

I was a Cub Scout watching movies of John Wayne killing Japanese during World War II, and as a high school student, I watched newsreels of MacArthur's and Ridgway's intrepid American soldiers slugging it out with the North Koreans and Chinese in the frozen hills of

Korea. I had read many books of military history, but what was life in the Army really like?

I mopped the sweat from my brow as I gazed around the Personnel Office in DeWitt Hall, on the north side of the Medical Field Service Quadrangle, Fort Sam Houston, Texas. It dawned on me, as I registered, that I was the only classmate wearing a suit and tie. I had donned them on that relatively cool summer day on 5 July 63 in Illinois to fly from O'Hare International Airport to San Antonio on Braniff Airways for $67.35, tax exempt. A blast of Texas heat and humidity slapped me in the face as I stepped off the airplane that day. This was my first taste of Texas climate: I had never been here before.

Billets, Classes, & Courtesy

After we registered, my classmates and I boarded an Army olive drab school bus. When our bus was filled, the driver, a corporal in starched fatigues and spit-shined combat boots, drove us out of the parking area to take us to the Billeting Office for assignment to the Bachelor Officers' Quarters (BOQ). We were chatting with each other, having no idea of where we were going, when we looked up to discover our driver had no clue about where the Billeting Office was; we were lost on the streets of Fort Sam Houston! During the course of our unplanned sight-seeing tour of the base, we passed through a residential area where oscillating sprinklers sprayed water on lawns shaded by stunted trees and shrubs. Small plaques planted in the yards announced the residents, Colonels and Majors, had earned awards for beautifying their lawns, which, in my opinion, resembled fields of homogenous blades of crab grass.

Bewildered and embarrassed, our driver stopped the bus, opened the door, and called out to two young men, dressed in civilian clothes, walking on the sidewalk, "Say, men, can you direct me to the Billeting Office?" One of them replied, "No. We are looking for it too. But we have a map of the base." When they boarded the bus, we discovered that they were our classmates, whose map reading skills led us to the Billeting Office on Wilson Road, south of the Medical Field Service Quadrangle, a scant two blocks from where we had boarded the bus about a half hour earlier.

In overhearing conversations among classmates seated behind me, I learned why the group at back of the bus lingered to retain spots at the end of the line queued at the desk of Billeting Office. Accommodations in the BOQ, for those of us unmarried, or who had left their wives at home, were fewer than needed, and these classmates somehow knew that if they were "unlucky" enough to be denied a bed in the base's Spartan quarters, bereft of air conditioning, they would have to *cope* with sleeping in the air conditioned comfort of one of San Antonio's motels, at government expense.

No Room at the Inn

Two of my companions and I failed to make the cut, but those behind us cheered when they learned there was no room for them on the base. But our billets were better than those of the men in front of us assigned to the BOQ. Mine turned out to be a single room with an oscillating fan and a bathroom, shared with a fellow officer, on the second floor of the Nurses Quarters of Brooke General Hospital at the north end of MacArthur Field. A stern looking armed guard stood in front of a roped-off hallway on the first floor, denying access to rooms occupied by nurses.

Our classes in the Medical Field Service School (MFSS) were held in buildings in the MFSS Quadrangle about a half mile to the south at the other end of MacArthur Field, a huge parade ground.

MEDICAL FIELD SERVICE SCHOOL (MFSS)

Before I left Chicago for MFSS, Captain Robin D. Powell, MD, my partner for the next two years, related an apocryphal story about an earlier class of medical officers assembled in bleachers at the edge of MacArthur Field to witness an effort to recruit doctors to volunteer for service in an airborne unit. Seeking to reassure potential recruits of the safety of his mission, an Army physician had parachuted from an airplane to land on the field in front of the newly minted army doctors. But after jumping from the plane, his parachute lines fouled, sending him hurtling toward the turf. The loud crunch of his fractured femurs, and his screams of pain, put off even the most macho men from volunteering for this exciting duty.

OPENING CEREMONIES

Deafening martial music, played by the U.S. Fourth Army Band from the balcony of the Post Theater, welcomed us MFSS students, their wives and children to Fort Sam Houston at 1215, Tuesday, 9 July 63. At the conclusion of a march by John Phillip Sousa, the theater lights came up to illuminate Brigadier General James T. McGibony, MC, Commandant, and his staff, as they filed on to the stage.

After he led us in the Pledge of Allegiance to the American Flag, General McGibony told us that we had entered our course at MFSS, designed to prepare us to serve as Battalion Surgeons in the Army, defending our country against the scourge of Communism throughout the world in the Cold War. Most of us First Lieutenants and Captains had no idea how hot the Cold War would become in Vietnam during our tour of active duty. General McGibony concluded his summation of the course work for the next two and a-half weeks with, "It's like baseball. You get out of it what you put into it." I never quite caught the analogy to baseball.

CLASSMATES & FRIENDS

As we were dismissed from our first formation on the sun-drenched asphalt quadrangle, I recognized two familiar faces. James Dahl, MD, had been my dissecting partner in Anatomy Class at The University of Chicago School of Medicine. After his graduation, residency, and fellowship, Jim practiced hematology in Marin County, California. Later, at meetings of the American Society of Hematology, Jim and I would reminisce about our tour at Fort Sam. I was grateful he shared his sense of humor to lighten the days of this sometimes stressful course. I had not seen my high school classmate, Peter Dyke, MD, since he left with his family when they moved from Iowa City fifteen years before. Peter had just completed his residency in Neurology at Yale Medical Center, and he was now a captain, like I was.

There were 720 men—physicians, dentists, and veterinarians—in our class, scheduled to last about three weeks. The next class following ours included the same number of students and covered the same course material in six weeks. When I asked why the difference in time allotted for each course, I was told, "The Army needs doctors on active duty now."

HISTORY

Only a few weeks after the Continental Congress established the U.S. Army in 1775, it appointed surgeons as medical officers to serve in the Revolutionary War. The U.S. Army Medical Service, directed by the Surgeon General, has been in existence since 1818. In 1863, it included the Medical Corps (MC, physicians), the Medical Service Corps (MSC, administrators), the Dental Corps, the Veterinary Corps, the Army Nurse Corps, and the Medical Specialist Corps. Recalling that the cavalry had, in 1943, dismounted to change their mounts from horses to tanks (armor), and airplanes (airborne), I asked what role veterinarians now played in the army. I was told, "They inspect the meat for the mess."

The Medical Field Service School (MFSS) was established at Carlisle Barracks, Pennsylvania, in 1920 to train army personnel. In the spring of 1946, MFSS moved to Fort Sam Houston as a component of Brooke Army Medical Center. From 1920 through 1 January 62, 214,174 students graduated from the program to serve stateside and overseas.

MILITARY COURTESY AND THE UNIFORM

Robin Powell had taken the course the year before me. He told me that although we would be taught military courtesy, how and when to salute, and where to attach insignia to our uniform, discipline was relatively lax. Professors in the three week course, he said, "…began their lectures with a dirty joke about Texas climate, complained that not nearly enough time had been allotted for the proper exposition of their subject, and dismissed the class early." This was not what I experienced. Things had tightened up!

Medical Service Corps Officers, jealous of young doctors who had jumped from civilian status to instantly outrank them, decided they would no longer tolerate physicians who appeared late for formation with uniform hats and insignia askew, with one trouser leg rolled up to reveal unmatched socks. Moreover, our teachers filled the whole hour of their lecture, dismissing us but a few minutes before the doors of Quartermaster Supply Building slammed shut in our faces.

Catching our breath, after running three blocks from the Blesse Hall classroom to Supply to obtain required uniforms and equipment, we found the Quartermaster stuck rigidly to his posted hours, leaving us to stand inspection the next day, berated by MSC Sergeants for failing to appear in proper uniform. When we complained to them about the Quartermaster's intransigence, the response of our tormentors was, "Stay flexible." This sequence led to frustration and depression for those who failed to appreciate Jim Dahl's humor referring to this "Catch-22" situation.

So we took our three crisp, uncirculated $100-bills—I had never seen a $100-bill before we were handed our officer's uniform allowance—and found military clothiers in San Antonio open and waiting to outfit us with uniforms appropriate to possible assignments in Panama, Puerto Rico, Thailand, Vietnam, Ceylon, Indochina, Eritrea, Philippines, certain South American countries, Hawaii, Formosa, and Africa.

GENERAL ARTHUR MACARTHUR (1845-1912)

Arising early, I showered, dressed in my summer khaki uniform with my Brasso-polished belt buckle, pinned my *U.S.* and medical insignia on my collar, put on my spit-shined black shoes, and caught the bus to the other end of MacArthur Field for breakfast in the mess hall.

This vast central parade ground was named for the father of General Douglas MacArthur (1880-1964), General Arthur MacArthur. Arthur MacArthur won the Congressional Medal of Honor for gallantry in the Battle of Missionary Ridge on 25 November 1863. Later, he fought in the Indian Wars (1866-1890), the Spanish-American War (1898), and in the Philippine Insurrection (1899-1902). He retired in 1909 as Lieutenant General, the highest ranking officer in the U.S. Army.

BREAKFAST

Breakfast, served from a steam table, was a modest 4,000 calories of grapefruit juice, scrambled eggs, bacon, sausage, hominy grits, American fries, baking powder biscuits bathed in melted butter and honey, and coffee. All of this sweated out of our pores to soak our starched khakis, as we stood in formation after breakfast on the asphalt quadrangle parade ground in the sweltering early morning (0830) Texas heat, with both temperature and humidity in the 90's. Dismissed and relieved, we entered Blesse Hall for our first class of the day.

INSPECTING THE MESS

Classes related to the organization of the Army, and its operation, were informative because of my growing interest in military history. But the class and instructor I remember best, after all of these more than 50 years, was the lecture entitled: *Inspecting the Mess*. Our lecturer, a physician in his late 40's, sported a well-trimmed thin mustache, appeared at the podium in his major's summer uniform of short sleeves, khaki shorts, tan wool knee socks, and plain-toed black shoes with brass buckles. His appearance reminded me of a photograph I had seen of one of General Bernard Montgomery's British Officers in the North African Desert, preparing to fight Rommel's Africa Corps. I expected to hear an English accent of our urbane speaker, but I didn't.

Of course, the *mess* referred to the kitchen and dining facilities, not an unkempt barracks. Our speaker began, "Do not make unscheduled white-glove inspections of the kitchen as one of your duties as a medical officer. The object is not to catch the cooks doing something wrong, but rather it should be to encourage them to take pride in their operation. And remember, there is a difference between sanitation and aesthetics. We all have to work together and get along

32

with each other in this man's army." He went on, "Be the soldier's advocate. Do not permit line officers to operate on the long-held myth that they can successfully wean troops from drinking water in the field. *Gator-aide* is good!" In this hour's lecture, I learned more philosophy than regulations.

Captain Marvin J. Forland, MD

Marv Forland was, in my opinion, one of the best residents in the Department of Internal Medicine when I served as an intern and resident at The University of Chicago Hospitals & Clinics. From New Jersey, he graduated from Columbia University Medical School, where his mentor, the renowned Robert F. Loeb, MD, of *Cecil & Loeb Textbook of Medicine*, dominated the teaching service at Columbia P.&S. (Physicians & Surgeons) Hospital. Completing his residency at Chicago, Marv was commissioned Captain in the Army Medical Corps, assigned to the Renal Research Unit, Brooke Army Medical Center, Fort Sam Houston, Texas. Snatching a moment between classes, I contacted Marv, who took me to lunch in the cafeteria of Brooke Army Hospital. After lunch, I accompanied him on ward rounds, a welcome interlude, reminding me I was a physician.

Burn Unit

Marv worked closely with the Army physicians in Colonel Moncrief's Burn Unit, nationally recognized for its innovative care of patients with severe body burns. At the time, burn patients suffered extensive fluid loss through their burned skin, leading to dehydration, irreversible renal failure, and death. But doctors on the Burn Unit had prevented this sequence by administering unheard of large volumes of intravenous isotonic solutions to replace fluid and electrolyte loss.

Silver nitrate was applied to the skin to prevent infection that would lead to more fluid loss.

We visited one patient with an 80% body burn who had received 10 liters of I.V. fluids in 24 hours. His kidneys worked well, producing normal undiluted urine (specific gravity of 1.010). This unfortunate enlisted man had been cleaning a latrine in a barracks at Fort Hood, Texas.

He had been cleaning a rusty metal urinal with gasoline and an electric drill affixed with a steel wire brush. Inevitably, sparks from the brush and drill ignited the gasoline, which exploded, severely burning the private, leading to his air evacuation to the Burn Unit at Brooke Hospital. The very next day, his replacement arrived from Fort Hood with the same burns, and the same story.

San Antonio

On another afternoon, Marv gave me a tour of San Antonio—in 1963, a city of 600,000 people. The population has more than doubled since then. San Antonio became the major military center of the Southwest. Located there, were Lackland, Brooks, and Randolph Airbases, and the premier Wilford Hall Air Force Medical Center. Shortly after joining the staff at The University of Iowa Hospitals & Clinics in 1969, I took care of an elderly patient from Illinois, for whom I had the difficult duty of telling him his diagnosis was acute leukemia. Without emotion, he replied, "That is the disease that took my uncle's life. He was a doctor and a general in the Air Force." In response to my query, he said, "His name was Wilford Hall, my mother's brother."

Now serving as home of the 4th U.S. Army Headquarters and Brooke Army Medical Center, Fort Sam Houston was established in

1879. Troops trained there for the Indian Wars, the Spanish-American War, World Wars I&II, the Korean War, and the war in Vietnam.

ALAMO (SPANISH FOR "COTTONWOOD")
As an Indian Village at the source of the San Antonio River, the region attracted Franciscan Friars from the Canary Islands, who founded in 1718 the first of several Spanish missions, San Antonio de Valero. Marv and I visited the only remnant of the mission, the Alamo.

We entered this historic church, the "cradle of Texas Liberty," on a hot sultry afternoon. An oppressive atmosphere closed in upon us. It was dark, cool, and clammy despite a slight breeze from an oscillating fan high on the ceiling. The Daughters of the Texas Revolution had asserted that a proposal to install air conditioning would desecrate the shrine.

Texas insurgents captured the Alamo from the Mexicans in December 1835. One hundred eighty Americans occupied it when General Santa Anna appeared outside the doors with several thousand uniformed, heavily armed troops, demanding surrender. Without reinforcements, William B. Travis, James Bowie (his brother, Rezin Bowie, invented the Bowie knife), Davy Crockett, and their men bravely fought their enemy against overwhelming odds in a fierce battle lasting from 24 February —6 March 1836.

In the end, all 180 Texan defenders were killed. Their martyrdom raised the battle cry, "Remember the Alamo." This inspired the Texas Army, led by Sam Houston (1793-1863), to defeat the Mexican Army six weeks later at the Battle of San Jacinto, assuring Texas independence. The State of Texas purchased the site of the Alamo in 1883-1905, and restored the shrine in 1936-1939.

Two thoughts struck me. A list of names on the wall of the Alamo showed that its defenders came from Tennessee, like Davy Crockett, and from other slave states in the southern United States. A blasphemous tourist from the north said, under his breath, "There would be no Texas if there had been a backdoor to the Alamo." For economic reasons, Mexico had encouraged colonization of its northern territories by Americans. But the Mexican Constitution, adopted after Mexico had gained independence from Spain in 1821, had abolished slavery.

In 1835, President Santa Anna extended the abolition of slavery to all Mexican territories. Settlers from America in that territory, later to become The Republic of Texas, seceded from Mexico. Ironically, rarely mentioned by popular historians, those colonists from the southern states of America, fought for independence from Mexico for their freedom to deny freedom to their slaves. In another twenty five years, the Texans seceded from the United States of America for the same reason.

ROUGH RIDERS

Later into our tour, Marv and I stopped for a moment at the bar of the Menger Hotel, a block or two from the Alamo. Here, in the spring of 1898, Lieutenant Colonel Theodore Roosevelt (1858-1919) recruited for service in the Spanish American War, The First Volunteer Cavalry; The Rough Riders. They were tanned-skinned cowboys and lawmen from Texas and Arizona, joined by a few blue-blood polo playing athletes from Princeton and other Ivy League Schools. Unfortunately, they had to leave their trusted mounts behind in Tampa, Florida, as they embarked in the transport ships for the war in Cuba.

Regular Army Regiments were armed with the new Krag-Jorgensen rifles, firing 0.30 caliber smokeless powder cartridges, while National Guard and other volunteer units carried the old "trapdoor," M1884 Springfield carbines and rifles that fired 0.45 caliber black powder cartridges. Teddy Roosevelt pulled strings to arm his Rough Riders with the new M1896 Krag Carbines.

Newspapers reported the Rough Riders' famous charge up San Juan (or Kettle) Hill, failing to give enough credit to young Lieutenant John J. "Black Jack" Pershing and his black regulars of the 10th U.S. Cavalry, known as the "Buffalo Soldiers." Their brave fighting, at the side of the Rough Riders, assured victory that day.

Teddy Roosevelt had raised the 1st U.S. Volunteer Cavalry after resigning his appointment as President William McKinley's Assistant Secretary of the Navy. Admitting his lack of military experience, Teddy deferred to Leonard Wood, MD (1860-1927), an 1884 graduate of Harvard Medical School, who accepted the post of Colonel of the Rough Riders.

While in the cavalry Wood had, with Captain Henry W. Lawton, left Fort Huachuca, Arizona, to pursue and capture Geronimo, for which Wood received the Congressional Medal of Honor. By December 1899, Leonard Wood had become the military governor of Cuba, and by 1910, Chief of Staff of the U.S. Army. During the convention in the campaign of 1920, he lost the Republican nomination for the office of the President of the United States to Warren G. Harding on the tenth vote. Fort Leonard Wood, Missouri, is named for him.

ATTITUDE ADJUSTMENT

After long hot days of classes, formations, and marches, Marv intro-duced me to "attitude adjustment" in the air conditioned Fort Sam's Officers' Club, which featured martinis for ten cents apiece. It was a nice way to end the day. Not the least of his generosity, Marv loaned me his broken-in black leather combat boots, so I did not have to suffer blisters from my new boots during my up-coming five-day assignment to Camp Bullis. Marv was slightly shorter than I (5'10" or 5'11"), of medium build, sandy hair, easy smile, an unflappable disposition, with fortunately my foot size, 10½ E. Marv made my 2- ½ weeks in Texas, not only bearable, but pleasurable.

Doctors Under Fire

"UNIFORM TREATMENT WITH M1960"

Several items in our mimeographed BAMC regulations deserve quoting verbatim:

> "5. Prior to dipping uniforms in the mixture all plastic items (watch crystal, ball point pens, glasses frames, etc.) should be protected from contact with the mixture (M1960 is a plasticizer and will damage these items)."

> "6. Fatigue jacket and pants are dipped in the solution one at a time. Thoroughly immerse each item and wring dry with hands. Do not place wet fatigues on the grass or on any painted surface (M1960 will kill the grass and remove paint). Pour any excess M1960 out on the pavement of the parking area."

Item 10 admonished us to dry the uniforms outdoors on a clothesline and not in a commercial dryer, for obvious reasons.

Item 11 said that we should not launder the treated fatigues, because that would reduce the "efficiency of the repellent." But uniforms "could" (read: should) be starched before pressing.

Pressing the pants with my steam iron released a familiar nauseating stench and sealed the surfaces together, requiring me to pry open the pants leg with a stick before donning the trousers.

I dreaded wearing these toxic, occlusive garments in the hot, humid days at Camp Bullis, but it probably beat being eaten by Texas ticks and mosquitoes.

Camp Bullis—The Mess

I could not have imagined a more desolate God-forsaken place to hold field exercises than Camp Bullis. My classmates and I stepped off buses, which had conveyed us on a sweltering July afternoon from Fort Sam to this wasteland of sand, scrub trees, and brush. An abandoned mess hall with corrugated rusting iron roof and concrete floor provided shelter for cots and our sleeping bags. For supper, we marched single file about a half block to line up at one end of a portable steam table and held out our mess kits to receive the army cooks' version of corned beef hash. After this wholesome tasty meal, we scraped remnants into one large oil drum and thrust our mess kits into another, filled with boiling water.

At dusk, several classmates had gathered around a bush near the sidewalk to our shelter. There, in the center of a beautifully created web was a large bulbous black spider with a red hour glass on its back, a Black Widow Spider. Indigenous scorpions gave us another reason to shake out our boots in the morning. One had stung a classmate on his heel, who was wearing thong sandals, raising a large painful welt. It was the first and last time I saw these formidable arachnids in the wild. I don't miss them.

Reveille

Reveille, followed by footfalls on the roof of our shelter, and a "thump" on the ground, awakened us the next morning. It was hard to tell whether it was Dr. Arthur Ahearn's gung-ho ambition to join the Rangers or just stupidity that led this former University of Chicago Surgical Intern to jump off our roof every morning, toughening himself for parachute training.

Medivac

Classes began with triage and evacuation of simulated battle casualties. We lifted groaning enlisted men, bearing wounds labeled with tags and attired in various red-stained dressings, on to stretchers. One "comatose" soldier with a bandaged head wound tightly shut his eyes until he winked and smiled at us. Each of our group of four grabbed an end of his stretcher poles, hunched over and ran to safety with our wounded man through high grass and shrubs amid the din of recorded machine gun fire and grenade explosions, broadcast over hidden amplifiers. At a clearing, we called on radio for helicopter evacuation of our victim. He waved at us from the helicopter as it ascended to take him from view. I think he survived.

Weapons Familiarization

By 1963, the venerable M-1 Garand infantryman's rifle of World War II and Korea had been replaced by the M-14, issued to U.S. and NATO (North Atlantic Treaty Organization) Forces.

A Major demonstrated its features as well as those of other pieces. The M-14 had a high capacity magazine, a tendency to kick, and to rise with rapid fire, features the Major did not want to trust us doctors to experience.

To demonstrate the shock on simulated human tissue of the famous, and not yet obsolete, Colt M1911A-1 semiautomatic pistol, our instructor fired its 0.45 caliber round into a block of gelatin at 20 yards. It exploded on impact before our eyes. Yet the smaller 0.233 caliber round, fired at a higher velocity from the new Colt AR-16 service rifle, did similar damage.

M-1 Carbine

Colt's M1911A-1 pistol was the sidearm usually issued to officers and medical personnel for their defense, but most officers preferred to carry the semiautomatic 0.30 caliber M-1 Carbine when in combat in World War II and in Korea.

Designed by "Carbine" Williams of the Winchester Repeating Arms Company, the M-1 Carbine performed well in service. Approaching obsolescence in 1963, it was light weight and had a longer barrel than the pistol, so our trainers figured we were less likely to shoot ourselves or our comrades while familiarizing with this weapon.

A Casualty on the Firing Line

While about 300 of our group sat in shaded bleachers observing the firing range, twenty of us occupied positions on the firing line. I enjoyed banging away at targets appearing at various distances down range. The M-1 Carbine was fun to shoot when it didn't jam. Our training arms, veterans of many previous classes at MFSS and elsewhere, had seen much service before we got them.

"Cease Fire!" the Range Master's voice came over the public address speaker as we waited in the bleachers for the last twenty of our group to complete their training. After a few seconds of silence, a loud *"bang"* focused all eyes on the far left end of the firing line to ascertain the cause of the report.

"I said Cease Fire!" the Range Master yelled into his microphone. A sergeant, standing with a student at the firing position of interest, raised a carbine in his left hand and waved his right hand saying, "I was fixing this jammed carbine. Everything is OK." But as he turned toward us, a red stain on the front of his white T-shirt the size of a saucer began enlarging to the size of a dinner plate.

Two MSC enlisted men let out a *"Woop!"* as they ran frantically to the sergeant. Another man, yelling at the top of his lungs, jumped in an ambulance parked nearby. He spun the tires, skidded sideways to a stop. The three grabbed the sergeant, protesting his wound was "nothing," and threw him in the back of the ambulance. They drove away, siren blaring, as 300 of us future battalion surgeons stared incredulously from the bleachers as this chaotic scene played out in front of us. At the Aide Station, the hapless sergeant underwent "surgery" where a corpsman extracted with tweezers a tiny fragment of a cartridge ejector claw from the jammed carbine that had pierced the superficial skin of his chest. Was this the kind of response serious injuries of troops in the battlefield might evoke, we shuddered to think.

Jungle Walk

A simulated "Jungle Walk," the next exercise, was scary. For each of us armed with a carbine, loaded with live ammunition, a corporal followed behind us a few steps as we crouched to walk on a narrow path lined with battle-scarred trees. Steel man-sized silhouette targets for us to shoot popped up at unexpected intervals.

It would have been great fun, except that I walked through the course with five classmates abreast, who had never before today held a firearm, and had no idea where they pointed the muzzle of their carbine. The corporal, walking behind each of us, dogged our steps, so he could deflect a shot that might pick off a young doctor instead of an inanimate target. His presence failed to relieve my insecurity of firing guns in the vicinity of those unfamiliar with handling firearms safely.

NRA

Congress cut spending for the military after the Civil War, so stringent budgets restricted army commanders from purchasing ammunition for target practice. But during the Indian Wars of the late 1860's and 1870's, it dawned upon officers that their troopers rarely hit what they aimed at. Realizing the need to change priorities, the army brass introduced target practice and marksmanship evaluations into the small postwar cavalry and infantry units.

Americans' reluctance to support a large standing army during peacetime meant that the United States would rely on civilians, inducted to the armed services, to defend their country during war. It took time to train fresh recruits to capably handle firearms so that they would shoot the enemy, and not shoot themselves. So, the National Rifle Association (NRA) was formed in 1871 to promote marksmanship and gun safety for civilians who would be called from their communities to defend the United States from foreign aggressors. The need for NRA instruction for civilians to be trained in the safe handling of firearms was graphically illustrated by my MFSS classmates, crouching in the next parallel line of the Jungle Walk, unsure of how to deal with the lethal weapons they held.

After World War II, a Japanese colonel was asked by a reporter why his troops had not invaded California after Pearl Harbor, in 1941, when Japanese ships and submarines were sighted offshore. He replied, in essence, "We knew that nearly every American household contained firearms of residents who could use them, and we dared not risk the casualties that would occur if we landed on California shores."

TRUST

To consolidate power over their lives, totalitarian governments disarm their citizens. In contrast, the American government serves at the pleasure of its people, and the Second Amendment of the Constitution of the United States of America recognizes the right of the individual citizen to own and bear firearms: "A well regulated Militia, being necessary to the security of a free State, the right of the people to keep and bear arms shall not be infringed." In the other amendments to the Bill of Rights (I, IV, IX, and X) the word "people" refers to persons.

Our Founding Fathers, including President Thomas Jefferson and President James Madison, and the courts, have upheld that the right to bear arms pertains to the person and not the State. It means that government officials must trust the citizen, who in turn, trusts his government. In countries like Great Britain, Canada, and Australia, when the government banned private ownership of firearms, violent gun-related crime increased dramatically while it decreased in America. Criminals kept their guns in Britain and preyed upon vulnerable unarmed citizens. In the year 2005, a citizen of Scotland was eight times more likely to be assaulted than a person in the United States.

CONFIDENCE COURSE

At 3:00 pm, a blazing Texas sun beat down on our group of 100 students, the first of three groups to walk the 75 yards of rock over which we were scheduled to crawl that afternoon. On the bottom of the mild slope, two M1918 Browning water-cooled 0.30 caliber machine guns, set to spray bullets four feet over our heads, pointed menacingly at us. Barbed wire, under which we were to wiggle, stretched between rusty iron stakes at intervals one foot off the ground in our path. It wound past craters containing explosives, planted to simulate exploding artillery rounds, fired at us during our passage through the "confidence course."

Our preliminary walk-through was designed to familiarize us with the terrain, but the unspoken reason that we did this was to shoo away rattlesnakes and scorpions which had selected our path on which to sunbathe. A rumor, propagated by MSC personnel, described a former student, who while crawling through the course in a previous exercise, encountered a diamondback rattlesnake face-to-face, stood up to avoid being struck, and was dispatched by overhead machine gun fire.

After the walk-through, we got down on our bellies, grateful for the padding of our elbows and knees, and for the protection of our tough army-issue leather gloves that helped us negotiate the barbed wire. A shrill whistle signaled the machine gunners to commence firing, and for us to start crawling. Sweating and stinking from the M1960 tick repellant in my fatigues, I squeezed under the first stretch of barbed wire, seeing very little, because my steel helmet obscured frontal vision. When I became aware I had sidled up to a crater with raised edges, its contents exploded with a huge "bang" spewing gravel and dust all over us. Despite ear plugs, the din of machine gun fire and of the periodic explosions was deafening.

Secure in the belief that the Army needed doctors, and that our trainers would not risk shooting us before sending us to the front, we struggled to reach the end of the course. Surely, the machine gunners were firing blank ammunition to simulate our combat experience. Nevertheless, the first wave of us to finish, cheered, confident we had not "chickened-out" under fire.

After completing the afternoon course, our First Group of 100 men collapsed in the shade of a grove of trees while we waited for our classmates in groups 2 and 3 to finish their course. We shared "war stories" during the evening mess about how we had fulfilled our mission while crawling under unrelenting machine gun fire. We chatted about possible future assignments, anticipating dusk, when we were scheduled to renegotiate the confidence course in the dark.

Sound Off

"You 100 men in First Group, form in one rank, and sound off!" barked the MSC Lieutenant. In the growing darkness, we stood in formation and sounded off: "1,2,3,...99, 100, 101, 102, 103." The lieutenant looked perplexed, then he said, "All right, gentlemen. Three of you are trying to sneak into First Group so you can finish the confidence course early. Now, you men in Group 2 or 3 know who you are, so step out of rank!" Again, First Group, sound off!" We did, "1, 2, 3,...99, 100, 101, 102." Silence followed. Then one member of First Group stepped back, proclaiming, "I'm a member of First Group, but I will not go through the course with a couple of cheats." Finally, the tension diminished when the third count ended with, "100." Silence followed. Then, after a moment of thought, the MSC lieutenant hopped into his Jeep with his sergeant, who drove him out of earshot so they could confer in private.

Military Justice

Returning from his conference, the lieutenant harangued us about honesty, integrity, character, and the ways a transgressor was rewarded, saying, "As a result of this childish behavior, First Group will go through the course last, after Groups 2 and 3." Indignant groans of injustice emanated from the First Group, since infiltrators from Groups 2 and 3 had perpetrated the miscounts. During our belated second trip under the rat-a-tat-tat of the machine gun fire, I looked up in the dark sky to see darting red lines of tracers passing four feet overhead. Someone said, "My God! They weren't kidding. They are shooting real bullets over us!"

Graduation & Leave

ASSIGNMENTS

When we returned to Fort Sam Houston, my classmate and neighbor in our billet, an unmarried First Lieutenant, was chagrined to learn that he had been assigned duty as a medical officer in Korea. This led him to pursue several hours of negotiations with the Army, after which he was ordered to report for duty at Tripler Army Hospital in Honolulu, Hawaii. That sounded like a cushy deal, but the catch was that he had agreed to serve three years' active duty in the Army, instead of two. Moreover, there was no guarantee that the Army would keep him in Hawaii for all three years.

My orders assigned me to WRAIR (Walter Reed Army Institute of Research), Washington, D.C. with duty station, Joliet, Illinois. So far, so good, but who knew whether Army Brass would change their minds about my assignment, depending upon circumstances that might arise in the months to come.

COMMENCEMENT

Student wives, cuddling their babies, their babies' crying drowned out by the martial music of the 4th Army Band, lined the back rows as we graduates in our smart new summer dress uniforms filed into seats of the Post Theater on 23 July 1963. General McGibony and his staff entered from stage right and led us in the Pledge of Allegiance as we saluted the flag.

He began a review of our course, anticipating our challenges in the months ahead, when suddenly, "BANG!" the power failed, plunging us into to total darkness. Air-conditioner fans whined down to leave us in complete silence. For a moment, no one uttered a word, then, undaunted by complete darkness and a dead microphone, General

47

McGibony rose to the occasion. In a ringing command voice, he complimented us on completing the course and wished us well. After his concluding remarks, we felt our way to the open back door that admitted outside light, and we filed out into the sunshine. Was the experience of these past three weeks a hint of what we could expect from life in the Army?

What We Learned

We had learned military courtesy, when to salute and how to wear our uniform. My certificate, dated 23JUL63 stated:

> "Students in the Army Medical Service Officer
> Basic Course (8A-C20A), during period 9JUL63 to
> 23JUL63 completed training as shown:
> 1. Weapons Familiarization
> 2. Battle Indoctrination
> 3. Evasion and Survival Training
> 4. Safeguarding Defense Information
> 5. CBR and Nuclear Training"

The motto of the Medical Corps, "To Conserve the Fighting Strength," really had greater meaning, I realized, when it occurred to me that a soldier was more likely to enter combat if he could count on being evacuated quickly from the battlefield to receive effective medical care for a wound in a well-equipped hospital, staffed by an expert surgical team.

Another thing I learned at MFSS, and during the next two years of my active duty, was that an Army unit is as efficient as any other group of people, depending upon the attributes of the personnel and the attitudes they bring to their work.

Reunited, 24 July 1963

What a thrill to see Karen and nine-month-old Bobby on the tarmac of the La Crosse Wisconsin Municipal Airport as I descended the stairs from the airplane that had carried me from Chicago's O'Hare Airport! Bobby had grown taller and started to stand and walk a few steps in the time I was in Texas. Earlier in the day, my Braniff Airways flight had left San Antonio at 7:30AM for Chicago with a transfer to Northwest Airlines to La Crosse. The flights had been on time, but the great desire to see my family during an up-coming three-day leave made the trip seem inordinately long. After hugs and kisses, Karen said, "I wasn't sure it was you." Despite a liberal application of sunscreen in the days preceding, my face glowed red, and a split lower lip was beginning to heal after blistering from exposure to the Texas sun.

GOD'S COUNTRY

To meet my plane, our good friends Charles and Lucile Price had driven Karen and Bobby from Decorah, Iowa, where my little family had been staying with Karen's folks while I was in Texas. Chuck drove us south from La Crosse on Wisconsin's Great River Road (WI 35) where I was overwhelmed by vistas of tall oaks and maples on bluffs reaching the water's edge along the beautiful Upper Mississippi River. The wooded islands, covered with green foliage in this the Driftless Area, contrasted with the dry scrub trees and sand of Texas I had witnessed. Although the temperature was in the 80's, a light breeze felt cool compared to the stifling heat and humidity I had left behind that morning. Indeed, this was God's Country.

After living in their basement for the last twelve years, Karen's parents were able to afford and complete their house in Decorah. It was under construction when we arrived, and scarce extra space limited our stay to overnight. So, the next morning Karen, Bobby, and I said goodbye, and drove east to our new home in Plainfield, Illinois.

Part II. Stateville
(1963-1964)

Prologue

Passengers on the train stared at my future father-in-law, Ernest A. Sivesind, as he returned home to Decorah, Iowa, after serving in New Guinea during World War II. It was his skin, yellow from taking the antimalarial drug, Atabrine, for many months. After a few weeks at home, the onset of chills, fever, and muscle pains led Ernie's family physician, Dr. Larson, to accurately diagnose malaria, a common occurrence in men returning from the Pacific Theater of War.

Because Atabrine (an erythrocytic schizonticide) killed the red blood cell stages, and not the liver stages (tissue stage schizonts) of *Plasmodium vivax*, the malaria relapsed when administration of the suppressant drug was discontinued. As a consequence, an intensive search for a drug that produced a radical cure of *P. vivax* was undertaken in the late 1940's. Clinical trials in U.S. troops during the Korean War (1950-1953) proved that Primaquine, an 8-aminoquinoline, was the optimal tissue stage schizonticide, curing *P. vivax* infections. There were minimal toxic side-effects, with one notable exception. Ten per cent of American black men taking therapeutic doses of Primaquine became anemic.

To discover the mechanism of the anemia, so it could be prevented, the Medical Research & Development Command, Office of the Surgeon General of the Army, supported studies of primaquine-sensitive red blood cells by medical officers assigned to the University of Chicago-Army Medical Research Project in Stateville Penitentiary. Investigators on this project, directed by Professor Alf S. Alving, MD, had previously demonstrated the therapeutic efficacy of Primaquine.

Results of clinical studies at Stateville, published in the scientific journal, *J. Lab. Clin. Med.* of 1954, showed that Primaquine caused a hemolytic anemia in which older red blood cells of susceptible persons were lysed (destroyed), producing a population with a shortened life-span comprised of young erythrocytes.

One of the medical officers assigned to the Army Medical Research Project in the 1950's, was Ernest Beutler, MD. Working with University of Chicago Professor Guzman-Barone, PhD, an expert on sulfhydryl (-SH) biochemistry, Ernie first demonstrated a biochemical abnormality in primaquine-sensitive red blood cells, decreased concentrations of intracellular reduced glutathione (GSH). Glutathione is a free radical scavenger that protects cells against oxidants, like Primaquine. He found progressively decreased concentrations of GSH in red blood cells as they aged.

Subsequent definitive studies by Paul E. Carson, MD, a Public Health Service Officer, and his colleagues, assigned to the Project, showed that primaquine-sensitive red blood cells were deficient in glucose-6-phosphate dehydrogenase (G-6-PD), a key enzyme in the aerobic hexose-monophosphate shunt responsible for generating GSH.[†] Incidentally, *Science* paper's coauthor, inmate Charles Ickes, was a nephew of President Franklin Roosevelt's first Secretary of the Interior, Harold L. Ickes (1874-1952), and was paroled in the 1960's to manage Paul Carson's research laboratory at the University of Chicago.

---

† Carson, P.E., Flanagan, C.L., Ickes, C.E., and Alving, A.S.: *Enzymatic deficiency in primaquine-sensitive erythrocytes. Science 124*:484-485, 1956.

These investigations were undertaken in a laboratory on the Malaria Project in Stateville's prison hospital by Army physicians who had faculty appointments (Research Assistant, Research Associate) in The University of Chicago Department of Medicine. They worked with volunteer inmate participants to initiate these studies, later pursued by other scientists in laboratories throughout the United States and abroad. Results of studies on primaquine-sensitivity led to a better understanding about how mammalian cells protect themselves from oxidant stress, and about how the body defends itself against malaria. The investigations at Stateville eventually opened new fields of study, like pharmacogenetics, biochemical mechanisms of cell aging, and inheritance of enzyme defects related to the epidemiology of *Plasmodium falciparum* malaria.

When I asked why the Army would finance studies of red blood cell enzymology, Dr. Alving, the director of the Malaria Project said, "We saved the Army's bacon! When the Soviets launched the first space satellite, Sputnik, on 4 October 1957, and the nation's educators were asked to defend science education and research in America, the Surgeon General was called to testify before a Congressional Investigating Committee as to whether the money in the Army's research budget was used to fund *basic* research. So the Surgeon General trotted out our discoveries about G-6-PD deficiency in primaquine-sensitive red blood cells, which proved basic enough to continue support."

Alf Sven Alving, MD, Professor of Internal Medicine, was Director of the Renal-Vascular Section in the Department of Medicine at the University of Chicago. For the twenty years, since its inception in 1944, he had also directed the Malaria Project, officially known as the University of Chicago-Army Medical Research Project at Stateville Penitentiary, Joliet, Illinois. Dr. Alving claimed that more leaders in academic medicine graduated from his program at Stateville than from most departments of Internal Medicine. Indeed, alumni of the Project included a College of Medicine Dean, four chairmen of departments of Internal Medicine, a department chairman of Pharmacology, directors of divisions of Hematology, and other professors of Hematology and Genetics at Chicago, Western Reserve, Michigan, Northwestern, Rush, Iowa, and at other academic institutions.

As a medical student, resident, and fellow at the University of Chicago, I shared with my classmates in the excitement of these seminal discoveries of red blood cell enzymology (G-6-PD deficiency) reported in the world's scientific literature by Dr. Alving's group. Some members of his group were my teachers, colleagues, and friends. So, no persuasion was required for me to accept an invitation to join this productive research group and fulfill, simultaneously, my armed service obligation.

At the time, in 1962, I had no idea my plan to study the biochemistry of blood cells would later lead to an intensive search for drugs to prevent and cure emerging strains of chloroquine-resistant falciparum malaria from Southeast Asia. But this is how I came to volunteer for the Doctor's Draft, receive my commission of Captain in the U.S. Army Medical Corps, and accept my assignment to Walter Reed Army Institute of Research, with duty station at the University of Chicago-Army Medical Research Project, Stateville Penitentiary, Joliet, Illinois.

In his book, General Palmer characterized those years I served on active duty:

> The period 1963-65 was one of the most tumultuous times
> for the United States in all its history, for these years saw
> American military power committed to a war in Indochina
> which was to divide Americans to a degree unprecedented

since the Civil War a hundred years before. Two presidents
served during these years—John F. Kennedy and Lyndon B.
Johnson.[‡]

Plainfield, Illinois

A warm moist westerly breeze rustled the green corn stalks and red-dened our cheeks as Karen, Bobby, and I alighted from our little red 1963 Dodge Valiant station wagon after an all-day drive from Karen's parents' home in Decorah, Iowa. What else should we expect in rural Illinois, but heat and humidity on this warm summer day, 25 July 1963?

Standing on a concrete slab under the roof of our carport, we looked north about 50 feet to our new home for the next two years at 70 James Street, Plainfield, Illinois. Our apartment, 3A, was on the southeast corner of a recently constructed two-story stone-sided building with six units, three up and three down. Second floor units looked out over a railed balcony.

To the west, beyond a wood fence enclosing the property, over the cornfield a block distant, a row of trees lined the banks of the narrow Du Page River as it flowed gently south to join the Des Plaines River and Illinois & Michigan Ship canal just south of Joliet, Illinois. These waterways joined the Kankakee River to form the Illinois River, which emptied into the Mississippi River above Grafton, Illinois.

APARTMENT 3A, 70 JAMES STREET, PLAINFIELD, ILLINOIS
Karen carried Bobby, and I carried luggage through the outside steel door leading to a hallway. On the right, our solid wood door, marked *3A*, opened to a carpeted brightly lit living-dining room contain-

---

‡ General Bruce Palmer, Jr.: *The 25-Year War, America's Military Role in Vietnam*, The University of Kentucky Press, Lexington, 1984, p. 17.:

ing our sofa, chairs, and tables, which the Army had moved in for us before I left for Fort Sam Houston on 4 July 1963. A good-sized kitchen, a utility area, two bedrooms, and a bathroom were tastefully decorated and provided closets with ample storage. Frank Bond, our friendly landlord and contractor, lived south of us on James Street. He had recently built this fine, quiet, clean apartment house, and fortunately we were the first occupants of Apartment 3A.

Plainfield, Illinois, a town of about 2,000 people then, was founded before Chicago was, but it failed to grow as fast as the latter. It has grown since we lived there, however. A 2011 road atlas lists Plainfield's population at 13,038. An extension from I-55, the old U.S. 66, runs southwest from Chicago to intersect U.S. 30, the famous transcontinental Lincoln Highway, running northwest from Joliet, to form a 90-degree angle with its apex pointing west on Main Street in downtown Plainfield.

We settled in Plainfield, because it was ten miles directly west of my duty station, and because my partner on the Project, Captain Robin D. Powell, MD, and his family rented a house in town, facilitating car-pooling and the weekly exchange of the Army Car to attend Clinic and pickup supplies at the University of Chicago. The high school was north of our apartment on James Street, and a couple of more blocks north, it intersected with Main Street where we found a grocery store with fresh produce, a hardware store with galvanized bins of nails and screws, a women's dress shop, and a nice restaurant, *The Clock Tower*. Farther north of downtown, was a large glass factory, owned by the Continental Can Company.

THE POWELLS

Robin D. Powell was the youngest, and the brightest member of the Class of 1957, in The University of Chicago School of Medicine, and

Henry P. Russe was the oldest. Robin became Dean of the The University of Kentucky College of Medicine in Lexington, and Henry became Dean and Vice President for Health Affairs of Rush Medical School in Chicago. Richard Moy, another of their classmates, became Dean of Medicine and Vice President for Health Affairs, The University of Southern Illinois in Springfield.

Dr. Horace Powell, Robin's father, had obtained his PhD in bacteriology under the famous William Welch, Dean of Johns Hopkins Medical School. Welch was one of Hopkins' "Big Four" (Welch, Halsted, Kelley, and Osler). The senior Dr. Powell, working with Eli Lilly & Company in Indianapolis, Indiana, developed some of the early sulfonamides, effective against bacterial infections.

Skipping a grade in high school, Robin Powell left his home in Indianapolis for 2 ½ years of premedical studies at Johns Hopkins University before entering medical school at The University of Chicago. I graduated from medical school in 1959, at age 25 years, a year younger than many of my classmates, and two years after Robin, but we were both born in 1934. During his internship in Minneapolis, Robin Powell met Julie, an RN Nurse Anesthetist, and they married. In 1958, Robin and Julie returned to The University of Chicago for his residency in Internal Medicine and fellowship in Dr. Alving's Renal Vascular Section in the Department of Medicine. Thereafter, he joined the Malaria Project, with active duty service in the Army Medical Corps.

Robin joined **George Brewer, MD,** in 1962, as Captain in the Medical Corps for two year's active duty in the University of Chicago-Army Medical Research Project at Stateville. George developed a field test (methemoglobin reduction) for G-6-PD deficiency, and he had conducted clinical trials in our troops in Korea, proving the test's efficacy in identifying the enzymopathy.

Dr. Alving's propensity to embellish with red ink the first drafts of George's manuscripts he was preparing to submit for publication, accompanied by Dr. Alving's remarks disparaging George's knowledge of the English language, added to other perceived insults, led to shared ill feelings. To show what he thought of Alf, who was short and obese, George presented him with a gift he had acquired in Japan on his way home from Korea, a squat black lacquer pot. Alf, appreciating its symbolism, displayed the pot on his desk where both could see it when they reviewed manuscripts together. When I replaced George on the Project in 1963, I wished him well in his new position, Assistant Professor of Genetics with Dr. James Neel, The University of Michigan.

Julie Powell's warm smile and gracious hospitality welcomed us to Plainfield. She was a proud mother of David (4 years), Amy (3 years), and Will (4 months), for whom she cared with firm love and the efficiency of a capable nurse. David became a surgeon, Amy a lawyer, and Will, a businessman. Julie's friendly, ebullient personality contrasted with Robin's quiet reserve and focused analytical approach to solving technical and social problems. However, Robin's love of baseball, and politics, and his dry sense of humor, lightened his serious nature.

THE COMMUTE

Having spent little time in a correctional facility, let alone in Illinois' Maximum Security Prison, former home to thrill-killers Leopold and Loeb, and Chicago gangsters like Terrible-Two-Gun-Touhy, my first day at work was memorable, indeed! Karen had pressed my khaki summer uniform to which I had aligned and affixed my silver captain's bars, gleaming brass "US," my medical insignia, and nametag. I canted to the right on my head, two finger-breadths over my right

eyebrow, a green overseas cap with captain's bars. Silver buckled ox-
fords, shined with high polish, like my thin black leather brief case. I
was ready for inspection when Robin, in his uniform, picked me up
in the Army Car, a M1960 olive drab Ford sedan, at 0745, Monday,
29 July 1963.

We drove north for several blocks on James Street to Main Street,
and turned right onto Lockport Road. Free of traffic, we sped east
past fields of corn and soy beans stretching for many acres on either
side of the road. Open car windows admitted fresh air wafting over
grasses glistening with morning dew. Songs of meadowlarks filled
the air. What a contrast, I thought, commuting to work a month
ago in four lanes of traffic on the Dan Ryan Expressway! Lockport
Road terminated six miles east of Plainfield at Illinois 53. Another
two miles south on Illinois 53, along the Des Plaines River, brought
us to Stateville.

STATEVILLE—THE GATE HOUSE

We turned right off Illinois 53 to enter a long tree-lined boulevard.
Beds planted with gorgeous blooming flowers graced its center and
borders. Ahead, we saw thirty-foot-high concrete walls, studded with
ominous looking guard towers. Several men in blue denim trousers
and shirts, names stenciled over pockets, tended the flowers and
mowed the lawn. Robin parked the Army Car, and we walked across
the driveway, passed a tall flag pole bearing our country's flag gently
flapping against a blue sky, and entered the brick Gate House.

Whereas Robin was greeted with smiles as we walked through a
metal detector, I was greeted by a couple of stern-faced uniformed
correction officers, who proceeded with a thorough search of my
body and briefcase. Catching a glimpse out of the corner of my eye,
I swore the officer who was patting me down, winked at Robin. I

was "fish," a new inmate. However, that morning was the first time, and the last time, in two years that I was searched before entering Stateville, the State of Illinois Maximum Security Prison.

Not finding contraband, the guards let us to proceed out the back door of the Gate House. We crossed a courtyard and driveway, enclosed by a 10-foot high iron fence, to the covered entrance of the Administration Building. This three-story brick structure was incorporated into the east wall of the prison, its roof extending slightly higher than the top of the wall.

ADMINISTRATION BUILDING

After climbing a curving concrete staircase to the next level, we encountered a wide hall crossed by a vertical frame of floor-to-ceiling steel bars. Sealed and repeatedly polished, the spotless concrete floor glistened in the rays of sunlight coming through barred windows. A uniformed guard inserted a large key into the lock of the gate in the bars, admitting us to another 50 feet of hall, enclosed as a cage, by more floor-to-ceiling bars in front of us. Next to the telephone switchboard on the right was the steel-encased armory with its several hemispherical gun ports and bullet-proof glass. When the gate behind us clanged shut, a second officer inserted his key into the lock of the gate in front, permitting us to walk out of the "cage" and into the hallway of the Administration Building.

I still have the 3"x 5" identification card made at our next stop. Instead of a prison number under my face/profile photograph, "7.29.63" appears under "DR RL DEGOWIN." On the back of the card is typed: "DR. RICHARD LOUIS DEGOWIN," followed by, "Whose picture appears on reverse side of this card is employed by U.S. ARMY (MALARIA PROJECT) at the Stateville Penitentiary." On the right is my signature, partially covered by my inked right thumb print, and on the left signed, "F.J. Pate/Warden." Robin said he would introduce me to Warden Pate later that morning. In addition to the Processing Office, where I had obtained my identification card, the Administration Building housed many other offices, the Officers' Barbershop, and the Officers' Dining Room in the basement.

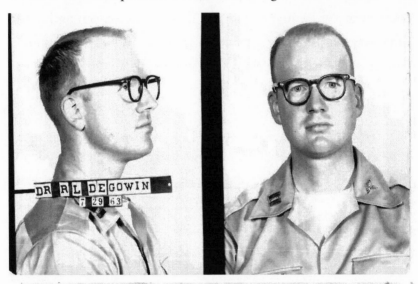

Identification Card, 29July1963

PRISON HOSPITAL

Robin and I walked east toward the hospital, past inmates in denims mopping and polishing the spotless hallway floors of the Administration Building. The 100-bed prison hospital was a separate three-story rectangular building, extending at right angles from the Administration Building into the Yard. It was connected by an enclosed hallway.

Dr. Julius Venckus, the full-time prison physician, occupied his office next to the dispensary on the first floor. The Diagnostic X-ray room was located across the hall from the Operating Rooms. Inmates from Menard, Pontiac, and the other prisons in the Illinois Correctional System were transferred to Stateville for major surgery and for treatment of serious illnesses other than tuberculosis. Two surgeons, practicing in nearby Joliet, were on call for help at Stateville. Two wards for inpatients occupied the second story of the hospital.

THE UNIVERSITY OF CHICAGO-ARMY MEDICAL RESEARCH PROJECT

An inmate ran the elevator, lifting us to the third floor of the prison hospital, entirely given over to the University of Chicago-Army Medical Research Project. Mr. William Messersmith, an ancient gentleman in a neatly pressed brown officer's uniform, arose slowly from a desk inside our unit and unlocked the gate with a key from a large bunch of them hanging on a ring attached by a short chain to his belt. In a Southern Illinois twang, he smiled and said, "Pleased to meet you Doc," and he shook my hand after Robin's introduction. Mr. Messersmith was not armed, as were none of the other guards whom I had seen—no firearms, no truncheons, no saps. His uniform, like those worn by all of the correction officers, had been made by inmates in the prison Garment Factory—his black leather shoes, in the prison Shoe Factory.

CONFERENCE ROOM

A long hall ran the length of the third floor from east to west. On the left were two wards, each with twelve white iron-framed beds, unoccupied and made up with clean white linens. Large south-facing windows lighted spotless rooms with sunlight. Beyond, on the same side of the hall, was another ward, now converted to a conference room containing a table, chairs, a large blackboard over a countertop of storage cabinets, and a wall-mounted television set. Doors to the two Docs' Offices opened off the end of the conference room. Each office had a barred window, like the rest of the windows in the building, built-in desks, shelves, files, and comfortable swivel desk chairs, an efficient use of a small amount of space.

Malaria Project Staff

THE OFFICE

Crossing the hall from the Conference Room, Robin and I entered a room through a door marked "Office." On my left, John sat on a stool at a draftsman's table drawing bar graphs representing Pyruvate Kinase concentrations in old versus young normal red blood cells. The inmate photographer, who had earlier that morning taken my portrait for the mug shot on my identification card, would photograph John's drawings and prepare projection slides for Robin's presentation at the Chicago meeting of the Central Society for Clinical Research at the Drake Hotel in November. He would also prepare 5"x 8" glossy prints of the graphs for submission to a scientific journal as figures accompanying a manuscript.

Over the next two years, working seven days a week with them, I got to know the eighteen inmates who comprised our staff on the Malaria Project. Most applied for their jobs with us after having volunteered to take malaria or having participated in drug trials, so they knew us, and we knew them. Their jobs required special skills, so we dared not risk spending time training men whom we might lose to early parole. Therefore, most of the men on our staff were doing hard time with long stretches for murder, armed robbery, or habitual criminality. Their lives before incarceration had not prepared them for their jobs with us, but, with few exceptions, the performance of their duties on the Project impressed me as superior or equal to that I had observed in life on the outside, before and after my tour at Stateville.

We "Docs," as the inmates called Robin and me, were not part of the prison's administrative staff, so some inmates spoke freely to us, as friends, about their past, some of which was public record. However, out of respect for their privacy, I have used fictional names in showing how men who had made mistakes in their lives—mistakes serious enough to require imprisonment in a maximum security prison—took advantage of opportunities to contribute positively to society, their chance for redemption.

John recalled for me his admission orientation to Stateville several years earlier. After encouraging his group of "fish" to serve "good time," Warden Pate called John aside to castigate him for disgracing his ethnicity. Of the more than 3,000 men in Stateville, there were only a few persons with Finnish ancestors, like John and Warden Pate. Unlike Warden Pate, John had blond hair, blue eyes, and a soft rotund figure. He, like the rest of our inmate staff, wore a white T-shirt, white cotton trousers, a black leather belt, and shoes, made in Stateville's Garment and Shoe Factories.

In his intake interview, the planned one-time meeting with the Sociologist extended to more sessions in her office when John dropped the fact that he had painted the walls and ceiling of his bedroom at home black. "She seemed taken with that, and it got me out my cell for a number of hours," he said.

John was taking to heart Warden Pate's admonition to protect his good name. John's lawyer was suing fifteen bar owners in Chicago under the Illinois Dram Shop Law, asserting that if they had refrained from selling John intoxicating beverages, which made him drunk and irresponsible, he never would have killed the man he was convicted of murdering. "It wasn't my fault," John claimed.

Danny, another clerk, was filing records in one of six steel four-drawer file cabinets, resembling those manufactured by *Steelcase* of Grand Rapids, Michigan. But in fact, they had been fabricated in the prison Sheet Metal and Furniture Factory. Danny transferred to our staff on the Project after serving as clerk to Assistant Warden for Discipline, Captain Pohlman. Danny told me Cap Pohlman was "firm, but fair." Moreover, Danny said inmates who cared about it, had the opportunity to complete their education, and/or learn skills equipping them for gainful employment after release from prison.

Cap Pohlman's full head of red hair topped a large muscular 6'6" frame that could easily intimidate a prisoner requiring discipline. This presented a notable contrast to his former clerk's diminutive 5'4" stature. However, Danny's striking black Irish features, honesty, intelligence, and work ethic, made him seem taller than his physical dimensions would suggest. He took advantage of his opportunity to work with us, and he later became an excellent research technician in our biochemistry laboratory. He told me that he was incarcerated for killing his nephew. I never heard him blame someone else for the crime.

Riley sat at a desk in the office typing Robin's letter to the Parole Board on an IBM *Selectric* Typewriter, a state-of-the-art electric typewriter, predecessor of computer word processors. Our letterhead, on good bond paper for the Army Medical Research Project, included my name. It had just arrived fresh from the prison's printing press. Riley's ability to recall from memory the names, numbers, and studies in which 180 inmate volunteers were actively participating was as impressive as his I.Q., measured at 148.

He had been born into a poor family in Iowa, hard hit by the Depression. Riley found his fortune in Chicago. There, he enjoyed his routine, arising at noon or later, and then frequenting the lush Chicago nightclubs, like *Mr. Kelley's*, to partake of great jazz, fine food, and good drinks. To finance this luxurious lifestyle, he stole diamonds.

Riley had infectious enthusiasm, a charming, likable personality, and the good looks associated with Irish politicians. I enjoyed talking with him. As time passed, with help from inmate technicians, he became an excellent biochemistry research technician in our laboratory, measuring accurately glycolytic enzyme activity in white blood cells and platelets.

I missed him after he was paroled. While I was out of town at a medical meeting, he came to our apartment in Plainfield one evening to see me. When Karen asked his name so she could tell me who had called, he said, "Tell Doc I'm doing fine. I am working for my uncle laying carpet, and just say Riley just stopped by to say 'Hello.' I used to work with Doc." Although I knew he meant no harm, Karen wasn't so sure about it when she realized Riley was an ex-convict. After he departed, she quickly locked the doors and windows, called Louise next door, and retrieved my old Colt 0.45 Revolver from my sock drawer, in case our visitor should return. I'm glad I identified myself before entering our apartment later that evening.

SHIRLEY HILL, RN

After the office staff had greeted me as the new Doc and returned to work, Robin and I stepped next door to the Nursing Station-Pharmacy. Shirley Hill dismissed the inmate working with her recording medications, shook my hand vigorously, and said in a hearty voice, "Glad to have you join us, Doc. Is Robin showing you the ropes?" Providing continuity as supervisor and registered nurse, Shirley, an attractive woman in her thirties, had seen Docs and inmates come and go during the eight years she had worked on the Project. She and her husband, Harry Hill, DDS, became our good friends. I came to rely on Shirley's experience, integrity, and good judgment over the next two years.

Shirley's blonde hair set off prominent blue eyes, and her starched white nurse's uniform covered a mature woman's full figure at about 5'6" tall in her white leather nurses' shoes. She had a warm smile, but she was tough, with a penetrating gaze, and the eighteen men who worked on our unit, doing time for murder, robbery, white slavery, and rape, knew that she would not take crap from any of them. They showed Shirley respect.

Shirley controlled access to our Pharmacy, for which Shirley, Robin, and I had the only keys. From there, she dispensed not only the usual medications found on any hospital ward, but at least seven different antimalarial drugs and toxic reagents used in the Chemistry Laboratory, next door.

The Chemistry Laboratory

Ed worked in the Chemistry Laboratory making timed precision measurements of enzyme activities in red blood cells with a Beckman Spectrophotometer, and measuring oxygen consumption of erythrocytes in a touchy Warburg Apparatus. His pre-Stateville experience for this job had been running the gross machinery of drilling rigs in the oil fields of Texas, and committing murder. Ed and his girlfriend had killed her husband with an axe.

On the wall above his laboratory bench, a framed document disclosed Ed's national board certification as a Medical Technologist. Indeed, this courteous and gentle grandfather, now trim in his mid-fifties, had used his many years in Stateville to obtain an education preparing him for a job requiring a skilled worker on his release from prison. With mixed feelings, I wrote a letter, detailing his accomplishments, in support of his parole. I hated to see him go.

Toward the end of my second year on the Project, Ed left us on parole for a job as a technician in the research laboratory of Dr. Robert Kellermeyer at Western Reserve Medical School in Cleveland, Ohio. Bob had preceded me as a medical officer on the Project by several years.

He knew Ed from working with him at the time. During a meeting of the American Society of Hematology several years after Ed's release, I was dismayed to learn from Bob that Ed had become depressed and reverted to alcoholism.

Working next to Ed in the Chemistry Laboratory as a technician, **Jean** had a French surname, but in his early forties, with the exception of his black hair, he hardly resembled my stereotype of a person of Gallic heritage; he was neither slender nor diminutive.

Most men on our staff had Irish, English, or German ancestors. None were Jewish or Asian. There were fewer than a dozen Jews, and only two or three Asian-Americans residing within Stateville's walls, home to over 3,000 men. There were no African-Americans on our staff, an ethnic group comprising about 20% of the prison population. Some blacks volunteered to participate in our studies, as had most of the men on our staff before we "hired" them, but I cannot recall one African-American applying for a position with us.

When Jean told me that he was incarcerated for "passing bad paper" (he meant writing bad checks), he did not explain why Illinois' Maximum Security Prison, which had no exclusively white-collar criminals, was his current home. When I asked him, "Why on earth would you pass bad checks?" Jean replied, "It's better than sticking a gun in a guy's ribs, ain't it, Doc?" Well, I was learning about a whole new relative value system.

The Hematology Laboratory

In addition to closely supervising our inmate nurses, and dispensing medications and reagents, Shirley spent several hours each day in the Hematology Laboratory. She and Robin taught me how to count malaria parasites, recognized from my sophomore course in Parasitology, on thick and thin blood smears of study slides. The three of us counted and confirmed the enumeration of the parasites by our technicians every one to four hours, or daily, as required by the circumstances.

Bailey—5 o'clock shadow, thinning hair, paunch, approaching age 60—took seriously, and with pride, his job as senior hematology technician and supervisor of a first class operation. Doing time for habitual criminality, more recently for running a white slavery operation in Southern Illinois, Bailey not only accurately identified and counted malaria parasites, but he performed hemoglobin and hematocrit determinations, and blood counts of white cells, platelets, and reticulocytes. He helped to train the other two hematology technicians, who in addition to the blood work, performed urinalyses in the lab. Kidney and liver function tests, and other special tests, were undertaken in the Chemistry Laboratory. Like Ed, he proudly displayed his framed certificate of Medical Technologist on the wall above his lab bench.

I'm sure Bailey wasn't ambivalent about receiving the grant of his parole after serving many years at Stateville, but I was. I was happy for him, and sorry for us, to see him go. His presence had been a mature, stable influence; he was a good lab manager.

One day, **Krause**—brush haircut, square face, trim body, early 30's—came out of the Hematology Laboratory, where he worked with Bailey, in a fit of pique, swearing, "Some son-of-a-bitch stole the candy bars I just bought at the Prison Commissary."

Krause just failed to see the irony. He was doing time for robbing grocery stores. It was not only that he enjoyed the expression on the face of the cashier when he approached her with a Luger pistol aimed at her heart, instructing her to fill his wife's grocery bag with the contents of the cash register, but there had been at least one time when he backed a semi-trailer truck to the loading dock of a Kroger grocery store and relieved the store manager of inventory. This lifestyle saved money on grocery bills for a while, until he got caught. He wasn't a *skinhead*, but he professed an admiration for Adolph Hitler and his Brown Shirts.

The other hematology technician, **Duncan**, told me he had a penchant for lying on a couch in the darkened living room of a house he had just burgled, waiting for the homeowners to return from an evening out, so he could terrorize them with his pistol when they turned on the lights. He was not doing time for robbery now, but rather for murdering his wife. Martha Jean, Duncan's attractive blonde twenty-two year-old wife, had been reported missing on Tuesday, 23 August 1960. According to William J. Brannon, on page 10 of the 15 November 1964 issue of the *Family Weekly*, under the title of "The Case of the Tasteless Killer," Duncan told the Chicago Police his wife had stalked out of the house the night before when he accused her of infidelity. The next day, fishermen found Martha Jean's body lying in peaceful repose near the Illinois River, dead from a single bullet wound.

The article continued to say that Detective Steve Coffey found no signs of a struggle or blood stains in Duncan's apartment. During his investigation, however, a young woman friend of the victim approached him, asserted that Martha Jean had been faithful to her husband, remarked that she was a wonderful housekeeper, and said, "That isn't the same rug that was here when I visited Saturday night. Martha Jean had excellent taste. She wouldn't have dreamed of putting a horrible thing like that in here. It clashes with everything in the room."

After failing a lie detector test and facing the evidence, Duncan confessed to shooting his wife with a rifle when she scolded him for having too many drinks Monday night after work. He had wrapped her body in the bloody living room rug where she fell, cleaned the blood from the floor, and disposed of her body. Then he burned the bloody rug and replaced it with a new one he bought for the living room, incriminating himself by making a poor choice of floor covering.

THE INSECTARY

In addition to the top floor of the Stateville Hospital, the Malaria Project had been assigned two large rooms in the basement, one for storage, the other for the Insectary. During our visit to the latter, Robin introduced me to a slender man, about 5'9" tall, clean shaven with black hair and a pleasant but penetrating smile. **Jerry** was bending over a low-power microscope dissecting the infected salivary glands of a female mosquito. He looked up, greeted me, and said, "Have a look, Doc." There on the slide under the scope were the sporozoites of the Vietnam (Sn) strain of choroquine-resistant *Plasmodium falciparum* malaria from Southeast Asia.

I began to perspire. A thermometer on the wall registered 82 degrees F., and a hygrometer showed the humidity was 75%. Jerry maintained this tropical atmosphere 24 hours daily, 7 days a week, summer and winter, despite the occasional breakdown of the air conditioning unit, which he ably repaired. He pointed to steel shelves holding separate white enameled pans of water containing eggs, pupae, or larvae, requiring daily transfer for breeding mosquitoes. One group of framed cages with tight mesh screening housed hundreds of adult *Anopheles stephensi* from India. Another group of cages housed *Anopholes quadramaculatis*, a local vector of malaria.

Jerry had worked on the Project since January 1963. He was conscientious, a hard worker, and master of his craft. He wasn't likely to be able to practice it after discharge, but that did not seem imminent. Later, Jerry told me that eleven years previously he had been assigned with eleven other convicted murderers to Death Row, for a murder he did not commit. He said all of his peers had been paroled or pardoned since then, but his "unfair" incarceration was perpetuated by his victim's family members appearing regularly at his parole hearings to protest his release.

Although Jerry claimed he was doing time for a "bum rap," he proudly described in detail to me how he had stepped out the back door of his house in Southern Illinois to place five well aimed shots from his Colt 0.45 Automatic into a prowler whom he said was stalking him. I gathered that murder never came to trial.

The Prison Community

Warden Frank J. Pate took the large cigar from his mouth, stood from behind a huge gleaming mahogany desk, reached over and warmly clasped my hand in a firm grip and said, "Glad to have you with us, Doc. Robin said you would be joining us this morning."

Although Warden Pate was probably no taller than my 6' height, this big solid man in his 50's seemed to tower over me. A man of few words, his presence filled the room. His black hair and eyebrows accented penetrating brown eyes behind black spectacle frames and a square jaw that commanded respect. Frank Pate had been at Stateville since 1939, when he started work as a guard under the tutelage of the legendary Warden Joseph E. Ragen. I was five years old then.

Warden Pate picked up a gray fedora hat that matched his pressed gray suit, pointed, and said, "Doc, this is Assistant Warden Revis (6'3", 300 lbs., wearing a black suit and tie), who will, with Captain Pohlman (6'6", red hair, brown officer's uniform), be making rounds with us, walking around the institution this morning."

EDUCATION

Our first stop was a classroom in the basement of the Administration Building. Inmates had the choice of going to school, obtaining vocational training, or working in one of the prison factories. "In addition to ensuring a safe and humane incarceration, our mission at Stateville is to prepare an inmate to return to society with an education and/or vocational skills, permitting him to earn a living without reverting to a life of crime," Warden Pate said, or in words to that effect. Even those men serving sentences of life imprisonment expected to get out. The new state law mandated that those men with a "life sentence" could appear before the parole board in 20 years, and in 7 years with "good time." An estimated 96% of inmates now serving time in prison would be released eventually.

At least 25-30% of the men on admission to Stateville were considered illiterate or functionally illiterate. Classes for grades 1-8, and classes for high school grades 9-12 (no chemistry), prepared an inmate student to take the General Educational Development Test (G.E.D.), leading to the award of a high school diploma by the Superintendent of Schools, Will County, Illinois.

College courses on television Channel #11 for the first two years, and given by visiting professors from Northern Illinois University at DeKalb, Illinois, for the third year, together with correspondence courses, enabled inmate students to work for a college degree. The average I.Q. (intelligence quotient) for inmate college students was 120. English was taught for Mexican, Cuban, and Puerto Rican immigrant prisoners, and a Criminology Course was offered by faculty members at nearby Lewis College. The Inmate Benefit Fund, the repository for income from the Inmate Commissary, paid course fees, tuition, and other expenses for education.

DINING HALL

It was about 10:30AM when our group left the Administration Building for our tour. We entered the Yard on a covered raised concrete walkway leading to the Dining Hall, a huge cylindrical building filled with chairs at long tables. Midday is traditionally the time for the big meal on Midwest farms, and a mouthwatering aroma of cooking beef, green beans, and bacon, wafted from the kitchen as inmate cooks in white starched uniforms and their supervisors prepared the big noon dinner.

Warden Pate addressed one of the inmates wearing a white apron and white paper chef's hat, asking, "How are you getting along, Jones?" He smiled and replied, "I'm doing O.K., Warden. Thanks for helping me get in touch with my sister." The Warden nodded, "You're welcome," and obtained a printed menu from him to show me. It listed the three meals of the day, including items available to inmates with special dietary needs and religious requirements. Prepared by a staff dietitian, the meals were balanced, varied, and contained ample calories. No inmate looked underfed or obese. With a good diet and plenty of exercise, these men were leading a healthy lifestyle—for some, much better than in their lives outside.

VOCATIONAL SCHOOL

Courses taught in the Vocational School provided inmates with opportunities to learn skills for jobs on the outside not easily replaced by advances in technology and automation. In 1963, computers and throwaway electronic devices were still in the future, so appliances needed repair to continue functioning. There were courses offered in repair of radios, television sets, office machines, and small appliances; maintenance of heating/air conditioning units, refrigerators; service of automobile engines; restoration of auto body/fenders; auto painting; welding; brick laying; machine shop work; sign painting; and drafting. Staff supervisors, and teachers visiting from outside technical schools, taught these courses.

An examination for licensing by the Illinois State Barber Board was taken by inmates graduating from the Prison School of Barbering. The school, in the basement of the Administration Building, boasted 44 chairs, fully occupied every day. Convicts were not allowed to wear long hair or beards. The room was brightly lit, and there was a hum of conversation and the smell of hair oil when one entered the Barber Shop.

I must admit I was a little anxious the first time an inmate barber cut my hair in the Officers' Barber Shop. Like a barber on the outside, he used a leather-strop sharpened straight razor to trim my sideburns. But for a professional haircut at 35 cents, I soon got over my concern and enjoyed chatting with the barber, whose prattle seemed no different from what I experienced outside.

TRADES AND INDUSTRIAL SHOPS

Leaving the Vocational School to tour the factories and shops, I paused to admire the tastefully designed beds of blooming flowers throughout the Yard. They were like those I noticed on the boulevard entrance to Stateville earlier that morning. After completing a 25-week course, administered by teachers from the Morton Arboretum, The University of Illinois, and the Chicago Park District, an inmate could obtain a certificate in Horticulture, Gardens, and Greenhouse. Convicts beautifying their environment here were learning skills in landscaping, increasingly in demand on the outside, and not replaced by automated technology.

Uniforms for officers and the clothes for the inmates were fabricated in the Garment Factory. A Textile Department supervisor taught the tailoring of the suits provided the inmates on their release from prison. Desks, chairs, and tables were manufactured in the Furniture Factory for the offices in Stateville, and for offices in other Illinois prisons and state institutions. File cabinets, steel desks, and duct work were fashioned in the Sheet Metal Factory. Inmates working in the Soap Factory produced bars of soap for personal use in the institution, and commercial soap used in the Prison Laundry. The Kitchen and Bakery cooks prepared meals thrice daily for about 4,000 persons—inmates and staff.

Skills learned in the Industrial Shops, Maintenance Shops, and in the Culinary Department might not be readily applied to jobs outside, but they saved the taxpayers money, contributed to the prison welfare, to the inmates' self-esteem, and kept the inmates busy with useful productive work.

The Honor Farm

Three hundred forty inmates, assigned to the Honor Farm of 2,200 acres, just outside the walls, cared for a prize dairy herd that produced 170,000 gallons of milk each year. They raised cattle, producing 475,000 pounds of beef, and hogs yielding about the same amount of pork every year. Truck gardens provided fresh produce, and men working in the Cannery canned 225,000 gallons of food in a good year. There were 95 bee hives on the Farm.

In 1966, the Physical Plant in Stateville had an estimated value of $100,000,000. That's impressive if you consider median home prices rose 10-fold from 1966-2006. It is even more impressive when you realize that these convicts, who had not led especially productive lives on the outside, could, working with the prison staff, sustain an almost self-sufficient community, larger than many small towns in Illinois.

Service

In a project of the Illinois Division of Vocational Rehabilitation, inmates sponsored by the Joliet Lions Club, recorded 230 books for the blind on 1,900 tapes. At this time, before transfusion-induced Hepatitis-B became prevalent and put an end to the practice, many inmates donated blood to the University of Chicago Blood Bank. Of course, they were not permitted to donate blood, if they volunteered for our studies of malaria and anti-malarial drugs, thus losing a stipend from that source.

For Body & Soul

The inmate teams, Trojans and Red Wings, hosted within the walls visiting baseball teams from Junior Colleges and other venues. In-house basketball games and weight lifting provided outlets for athletes and for others keeping fit. Meetings of Alcoholics Anonymous

(AA) were attended by many, and religious services were offered by in-house chaplains and visiting ministers, priests, and rabbis. Lutheran, Episcopal, Jewish, Baptist, Greek Orthodox, Roman Catholic, Protestant and Christian Science services were held regularly. Faith-based and other self-help programs attracted a number of inmates.

The Panopticon

In her 2007 biography of Aaron Burr, *Fallen Founder*, author Nancy Isenberg describes a visit of Aaron Burr, during his self-imposed exile in England in 1808, to the home of a political and social reformer, Jeremy Bentham. Bentham, the originator of *Utilitarianism*, proposed a new kind of penitentiary, the *Panopticon*, a cylindrical cell house. Isenberg's description of this, on page 374, could serve as a blueprint for the cell blocks constructed at Stateville in the 1930's.

Cell Blocks

Covered walkways, like spokes, emanated from the Dining Hall to five cell blocks, four huge cylindrical buildings, like the Dining Hall, and one newer long rectangular structure. As the wardens and I entered one of the round cell houses, I was impressed by the polished concrete floor, from which arose a central pylon guard tower and 4 galleries of 62 cells each, home to 570 convicts. An unarmed guard in the tower, four stories high, looked into each pie-shaped cell, designed to accommodate two inmates, and a third or fourth, until the new state law took effect, relieving the crowding by releasing 420 inmates in October. But in July of 1963, Stateville housed from 3,000 to 4,000 prisoners, crowded into five cell blocks, Segregation, Isolation, and on the Honor Farm.

If a violent outbreak occurred in a round cell house, armed guard reinforcements could be rushed there from the Administration Building.

Within the enclosed entrance on the second floor, "The Cage," fire-arms obtained in the Armory could be taken down an isolated stairs to a tunnel under the covered walkway to the Dining Hall, then through another tunnel under a walkway to a round cell house beneath the central guard tower and up the inside of the tower to the observation control area of the guard house. During our tour, and for the remaining two years that I worked at Stateville, I never saw a guard, officer, or staff person with a firearm, or any other weapon.

CLOSE CONTROL

After working for six years (1957-1963) as Sociologist for the Stateville Parole Board, Nathan Kantrowitz wrote: *Close Control: Managing a Maximum Security Prison.*[§] In his book, he tells us how Warden Joseph Ragen, from 1942-1961, turned Stateville from a chaotic institution, run by gangs of inmates and complicit guards, into a prison controlled by the Warden and his lieutenants. In 1961, Ragen's former assistant, Frank J. Pate, the new warden, continued "close control" of Stateville, in which tightly enforced discipline of both inmates and guards meant an inmate could do time without being beaten by fellow inmates or by a sadistic guard; there was no brutality, and no guard carried a gun or club. It was under these conditions that the research by medical officers and inmates could be safely undertaken for twenty-five years on the Malaria Project.

JAKE & LOUISE

Managing the start-up of a new glass factory in Montgomery, Alabama, was the last assignment Jake Kahler undertook before he retired in early 1963 from Hazel-Atlas Glass Company of Wheeling, West Virginia. But here were Louise and Jake Kahler, both about the

---

§ Harrow & Heston, Albany, NY,1996, pp217

same age of my parents, in their mid-60's, our next door neighbors in Apartment 2A, 70 James Street, Plainfield, Illinois. How did that come about?

Continental Can Corporation of America executives found that the eleven glass factories they had acquired from Hazel-Atlas were losing money, especially the glass plant in Plainfield, Illinois. They were able to divest themselves of ten glass plants, but potential buyers were reluctant to acquire the factory in Plainfield. To their credit, the corporate officers at Continental Can realized their people knew how to make cans, but they didn't know how to make glass. So they hired Jake, an experienced engineer and manager, to take over the Plainfield operation, hoping he could recover sufficient productivity to make the plant attractive to a buyer.

We became good friends of Jake and Louise, and during one of our social hours and dinners with them, Jake invited Karen and me to tour the glass plant with him. On the appointed weekend, Jake appeared at our door in a gray suit, tie, vest, and shined black shoes. He drove us northeast of town to the huge glass factory, its towering ventilators emitting heat waves visible from Interstate 55, several miles to the southeast.

The heat and white hot molten glass in the furnace reminded me of the Inland Steel Company plant in Indiana Harbor, which I had toured with my medical school class. Glowing red hot beer bottles popped out of molds onto conveyor belts at a rate of 130 per minute. *Aunt Jemima* syrup bottles appeared like magic out of molds in another area. Rarely, a beer bottle exploded on touching the conveyor belt. Pointing to the bottle's remnants, Jake said, "That's one reason Continental Can lost money. I found that the bottles exploded, because the temperatures of the glass in the molds were not homogeneous. They were uneven, because some of the molten glass in the furnace had cooled in pools before being poured into molds. Now that we drain those pools to remove the cooler glass from the molds, we have nearly solved the problem."

In a few months, Jake and his workers increased production, the glass plant made a profit, and the Kerr Glass Company bought the Plainfield plant from Continental Can. Mrs. Kerr, the new owner, practiced her faith. After planned infrequent interruptions in 24/7 continuous production, for maintenance and Christmas, she presided over the firing up of the glass plant's furnace with a religious service, attended by her manager and other employees. Jake said that somehow she had overcome her reservations about facilitating the consumption of alcoholic beverages and continued to make beer bottles at 130 per minute.

COMMUNISM AND THE COLD WAR

By 1963, most Americans finally realized that Russian Communism posed a real threat to the free world. As early as World War II, Great Britain's Winston Churchill warned President Franklin Roosevelt of the duplicity of our "ally," Soviet Russia's Premier Joseph Stalin (1879-1953), a ruthless dictator who had murdered millions of his own people to consolidate power in the purges of the 1930's. Yet, as if he didn't take Stalin seriously, Roosevelt referred to him as "Uncle Joe."

For worldwide Communism to prevail, according to Vladimir Lenin and the Soviet leaders, violent overthrow of democratically elected governments would be necessary, a position endorsed by the American Communist Party. To believe the myth, accepted by liberals and Communists, like Alger Hiss, in the Roosevelt Administration, that the "state would wither away" once Communism was accepted worldwide, was silly. Like Fidel Castro of Cuba, no leader of a recent "people's" revolution, ever gave up power. Remarkably, in February

2008, after 50 years in power, 81 years old and an invalid, Fidel announced he had turned over his dictatorship to his brother, Raul, still retaining control. I cannot recall hearing of an instance of a powerful leader stepping down since that of George Washington, who willingly relinquished power and returned to Mount Vernon, after serving two terms as our first president.

VIETNAM

Taking heat from Republicans in Congress, who alleged he stood aside when Mao Zedong (1893-1976) and his communists took over China in 1949, President Harry S. Truman sent the Army under General Douglas MacArthur, whom he later fired, to oppose North Korea's invasion of democratic South Korea when Communist Troops crossed the 38th Parallel on 25 June 1950.

Just prior to the North Korean Communist aggression, Truman announced on 1 May 1950 that United States would supply aid in the form of U.S. Military Advisors to the French, clinging to control of their colonies in Indochina, Vietnam. President Dwight Eisenhower, who terminated the combat in Korea in 1953, felt he could not support French colonialism, and decided against armed intervention, but he continued to deploy a small group of military advisors in Vietnam. Communist Vietnamese forces defeated the French at Dien Bien Phu in May 1954, and Vietnam was split at the 17th Parallel in July of that year.

Ngo Dinh Diem, an autocratic Catholic ruler who became Premier of South Vietnam, set about to rid his country of the French and suppress the insurgent Viet Cong. Departure of the French in 1957 left a vacuum of military strength, which Eisenhower was reluctant to support with more than a small number of advisors; the Military Assistance Advisory Group (MAAG). However, General Edward G. Lansdale (CIA) and Presidential Assistant General

Maxwell G. Taylor, convinced President John F. Kennedy to expand U.S. Military presence in South Vietnam. After Kennedy took office in 1961, he increased troops from 900 advisors to 17,000 soldiers by 1963. Rumors in Saigon that Diem might negotiate peace with the North Vietnamese to free himself from the presence of American military personnel were unacceptable to President Kennedy after the loss of Laos to the Communists in 1961, when he thought he needed to hold free territory until after his anticipated re-election in 1964.

U.S. COMMITMENT IN VIETNAM

President Kennedy regretted Diem's failure to beat the Viet Cong, and JFK was politically embarrassed by Diem's brother Nhu's repression of Buddhist monks, who, in protest, doused themselves with gasoline and set themselves on fire in the street in front of U.S. press photographers. Following a military coup and the assassination of Diem and his brother on 2 November 1963 (blamed on JFK and the CIA), the Johnson Administration escalated the war in Vietnam with the further buildup of U.S. Military Forces in Southeast Asia.

Once again, American troops, after fighting the Japanese in the Pacific Theater of War during World War II, and fighting North Korean and Chinese Communists during the Korean War, were exposed to tropical diseases, like malaria. But this time, recent reports suggested that falciparum malaria in Southeast Asia had become resistant to Chloroquine, the mainstay drug that had cured the disease for the last 15 years.

Malaria ("bad air") and its Vector

Insecticides (DDT) and treatment of infected persons wiped out malaria in the United States during World War II, but in 2005 the

World Health Organization officials estimated that about 300 million persons living in 91-100 countries (80% in Africa, the rest in Asia and Latin America) were infected with malaria. Non-immune children became victims most frequently, with about 1.5 million deaths each year, mainly from cerebral malaria, caused by *Plasmodium falciparum*. Two of the four types of plasmodia which infect human beings, i.e., *P. vivax* and *P. falciparum*, account for most cases with rare reports of infections with *P. ovale* or *P. malariae*. Anopheline mosquitoes capable of carrying malaria, like our *Anopheles quadrimaculatus*, live in the United States, thus the fine mesh screens on our barred insectary windows and the handy fly swatters hanging on the wall. A reservoir of infected persons, upon which the mosquito vector feeds, is required to sustain endemic malaria.

LIFE CYCLE

A female anopheline mosquito requires a blood meal to lay her eggs. When she bites a patient with malaria, she ingests the sexual forms of the parasite in the blood she aspirates with her proboscis; macrogametocytes and microgametocytes. Unlike his vampire mate, the male's proboscis is not long enough to penetrate human skin deep enough to draw blood. In her stomach, the microgametocyte exflagellates to fertilize the macrogametocyte, which, in turn, forms an ookinete that penetrates the midgut wall to produce an oocyst. The oocyst undergoes sporogony (cell division) and ruptures to release sporozoites that infest her salivary glands. So the female mosquito releases with her saliva sporozoites into the blood of her next victim.

Sporozoites travel in the blood of the victim, penetrate liver cells, and mature to hypnozoites (or cryptozoites). In the liver they undergo exoerythrocytic schizogony (cell division) and are released back into the blood as merozoites where they attach to receptors on red blood cells. There they divide (erythrocytic schizogony) to form more merozoites to go on and invade more red blood cells. A small number form gametocytes.

THE INFECTIONS

Important differences in *P. vivax* and *P. falciparum* require different modes of prevention and treatment. *Plasmodium vivax* is less virulent than *Plasmodium falciparum*, but more persistent.

Plasmodium vivax parasites infect only the young red blood cells with the minor Duffy blood type antigen, which serves as the receptor for the vivax merozoite. Most black persons do not carry the Duffy receptor on their red cells, so they resist infections by *P. vivax*. Because vivax parasites infect only young red blood cells, parasitemia in non-immune white persons is relatively low (20,000-30,000/ul), so the acute attacks are limited. However, clearing the blood with a clinical suppressive drug, like Atabrine, does not cure the infection, because an attack with parasitemia may happen months or years later from retained liver stage vivax hypnozoites, and "relapse" is said to occur.

Plasmodium falciparum parasites infect red blood cells of all ages without requiring the Duffy receptor, so, with no suppression, parasitemia may reach high levels (>500,000/ul) in non-immune persons of any race. It can cause disseminated intravascular coagulation (DIC, consumption coagulopathy); blood clots in small blood vessels, ischemia, and organ damage. However, killing the erythrocyte (red blood cell) stages of *P. falciparum* infections cures the disease; "radical cure." But, if the parasites are suppressed below the level of detection, and not eliminated with a suppressive drug, and parasitemia with fever recurs within days or a week of stopping the drug, "recrudescence" is the term used to describe the attack.

Formerly, Chloroquine killed the blood stages of both vivax and falciparum malaria, and Primaquine killed the liver stages of vivax malaria. The recent emergence of chloroquine-resistant strains of falciparum malaria in Southeast Asia led to new challenges in the prevention and treatment of our troops exposed to malaria in Vietnam.

REVERSE BIOLOGICAL WARFARE

From extensive experience in the Pacific during World War II, it was abundantly clear to line officers and the Surgeon General of the U.S. Army that febrile soldiers suffering from attacks of malaria were ineffective troops.

Japanese occupation of the cinchona plantations in Southeast Asia in World War II guaranteed their military forces supplies of the cinchona alkaloid, quinine. Denied access to that antimalarial drug, American servicemen relied on the synthetic Atabrine (Quinacrine, Mepacrine), somewhat more effective as a clinical suppressive of *P. vivax* than quinine.

So, in the Pacific Theater of Operations during World War II, better antimalarial prophylaxis and treatment meant that Americans could put more healthy troops on the line in an endemic area of malaria than the enemy could—a form of "reverse biological warfare."

CHLOROQUINE-RESISTANT PLASMODIUM FALCIPARUM MALARIA

Isolated reports of the resistance of falciparum malaria to Chloroquine and other antimalarial drugs in patients treated in South America and in Southeast Asia appeared in scientific publications as early as 1961-1963. President Kennedy's deployment of more troops in Vietnam challenged Army Medical Officers to find ways of protecting and curing our servicemen of infections from a potentially lethal disease.

So within the year I had volunteered for the Doctor's Draft and reported for active duty in the Army, the emphasis in research at the University of Chicago-Army Medical Research Project shifted from studying arcane erythrocyte enzymology, related to drug-induced hemolytic anemia, to characterizing the drug-resistant strains of falciparum malaria from Southeast Asia, critical to finding prophylaxis and a cure.

VIET-NAM (SN) STRAIN

Research aimed at discovering the spectrum of drug resistance of the Viet-Nam (Sn) strain of *Plasmodium falciparum* was underway when I joined the Malaria Project in 1963; Powell, RD, Brewer, GJ, DeGowin, RL, & Alving, AS: *Studies on a strain of Chloroquine-resistant Plasmodium falciparum from Viet-Nam,* Bulletin World Health Organization, 31: 379-392, 1964.

Marine Captain Sn., a 34 year-old Caucasian, had been stationed for about one year near Nha Trang, Republic of Vietnam. Despite taking orally 300 mg of Chloroquine base every week to prevent malaria, he experienced an acute attack of malaria, and on 27August1962, asexual erythrocytic forms (merozoites) of *Plasmodium falciparum* were detected in a microscopic examination of thick smears of his blood. In the last week of August, recrudescence of malaria followed a standard therapeutic course of Chloroquine tablets (1,500 mg base over 3 days), and greater than standard courses of Chloroquine administered in September and in October failed to induce radical cure of his infection. Two weeks after the third course of Chloroquine, the patient was transferred to the United States Naval Hospital, Great Lakes, Illinois, where his fever recurred, and blood smears revealed *P. falciparum* parasites.

Studies of this strain of malaria were initiated on 1November1962 by inoculating infected blood from Captain Sn. into non-immune inmate volunteers on the Army Medical Research Project, Stateville Penitentiary. Radical cure of Captain Sn's infection was finally achieved by administering intravenously 1935 mg of quinine sulfate daily for 10 days, concurrently with 50 mg of Pyrimethamine daily for 3 days. In subsequent studies with volunteer inmates on the Malaria Project, it became clear that this strain of malaria was multi-drug resistant to standard previously curative courses, not only of Chloroquine, but of Hydroxychloroquine, Amodiaquine, Atabrine, Proguanil (Paludrine), and a new repository form of a proguanil metabolite, CI-501. Radical cures of the volunteers' infections were achieved with the administration of intravenous quinine sulfate for 10 days and Pyrimethamine orally for 3 days.

Sensitivity to Quinine

Unlike another strain of drug-resistant falciparum malaria from Southeast Asia, the Thailand (JHK) strain, in which a "curative" course of Chloroquine temporarily cleared the blood of parasites, followed by recrudescence, the parasitemia of the Viet-Nam (Sn) strain resisted suppression by a standard course of Chloroquine. Interestingly, the Thai (JHK) strain of drug-resistant falciparum demonstrated exceptionally increased sensitivity to quinine.

Two questions emerged: 1. Do other strains of falciparum malaria from Southeast Asia exhibit spectra of drug resistance identical to the Viet-Nam (Sn) strain? And 2. Could medical officers depend upon courses of quinine or Pyrimethamine to cure troops in the field infected with multi-drug resistant malaria? "No," proved to be the answer to both questions.

The Malayan (Camp) strain of falciparum malaria proved to be resistant to Pyrimethamine and every other antimalarial drug, except quinine, to which it was quite sensitive, and "no," officers could not rely on using quinine in the field, because the Army's supplies had been depleted to a total of 9,000 ounces of quinine, and half of that had just been sold. Fortunately, the Government reneged on its contract and recovered the precious quinine sulfate, a drug no longer produced by pharmaceutical companies. Clearly, the Army's stores of quinine were insufficient to treat the large number of soldiers expected to be deployed in the malarious areas of Vietnam, but the stores of quinine were sufficiently large enough for us to safely carry out studies to find prophylaxis and a cure for these mutated strains of multi-drug resistant falciparum malaria.

The Need to Use Volunteers for Studies

Investigators at the National Institute of Health (NIH) reported favorable responses to cycloguanil pamaoate (CI-501), a repository preparation of a hydrotriazine metabolite of chlorguanide, in mice infected with *Plasmodium berghei* (mouse malaria), in rhesus monkeys infected with *Plasmodium cynomolgi* (monkey malaria), and in other animal malarias. Cycloguanil pamoate, however, failed to cure infections of multi-drug resistant *Plasmodium falciparum* in volunteer inmates on the Malaria Project at Stateville. So testing potentially curative antimalarial drugs in animals with malaria was not an option, because responses in lower animals were not predictive of responses in human beings. Moreover, attempts to culture parasites *in vitro* for testing drugs met with failure. Thus, the necessity to study volunteers with malaria in the search for new curative and preventive medications.

Before the discovery of penicillin, doctors successfully treated patients with the insanity of tertiary syphilis by giving them malaria to produce fevers, signifying that the body's immune system would kill the infectious agent of the disease, the spirochete, *Treponema pallidum*. Quinine, and potentially effective antimalarial drugs used to control the malaria, were studied, but the concomitant illnesses and the poor health of the patients made it impossible to draw accurate conclusions about the efficacy and side-effects of the new drugs. So, when our troops were deployed, during World War II, in areas of endemic malaria, healthy non-immune inmates in the NIH program in the Federal Prison in Atlanta, Georgia, and in the University of Chicago-Army Medical Research Project in Stateville were permitted to volunteer for studies undertaken in tightly controlled safe conditions.

The Volunteers

Robin was engaged in other projects, so Dr. Alving and he assigned me to determine the spectrum of drug resistance, leading to prevention and cure of the Malayan (Camp) strain of *Plasmodium falciparum*. A twenty-three year-old, Private Campbell in the Commonwealth Forces, was ordered to the Thai-Malayan border, where he contracted chloroquine-resistant falciparum malaria in late 1962. Repeated treatment with several different antimalarial drugs failed to cure his infection, when in 1963, a course of intravenously administered quinine sulfate finally led to radical cure of his malaria. His infected red blood cells were used to initiate our studies at Stateville.

Inmates responded to bulletin board notices, and the prison grapevine, to volunteer for the proposed studies of the Camp strain. A volunteer had to be trustworthy to serve on a hospital ward, "up front," and have the proper attitude to cooperate with the physicians and nurses responsible for his medical care. After Warden Pate approved the applicants, eighteen men visited our unit, gathering in the Conference Room of the Malaria Project.

For each applicant, Robin and I took his history, performed a complete physical examination, obtained complete blood counts and urinalysis. We examined the blood smears, urinary sediments, and chest x-ray of each man who wished to volunteer. Tests of his liver and kidney function were performed in our chemistry laboratory. Our thorough diagnostic examinations assured us that these strong healthy young men in their 20's and 30's had no underlying illness that might impair their ability to tolerate the early stages of malaria or the side-effects of antimalarial drugs or other necessary medications.

INFORMED CONSENT

Of the 18 men who applied, we accepted 12 for the studies after determining they had completely normal diagnostic examinations. When we reassembled in our Conference Room, we explained to them in detail the reasons for the studies and the risks involved in participating. We told them we would stop the study and cure them of malaria, if they asked us to, or if we as physicians felt there was any reason to stop, at any time during the study. Then we answered their questions, but most of the men had spoken with fellow inmates who had volunteered for previous studies and knew what to expect.

We told the inmates if they had reservations about volunteering to withdraw their applications. If they took malaria, they would not be allowed to donate blood to the blood banks, so they could not receive the attendant stipend to spend in the Commissary. On completion, Robin or I would write a letter recognizing their participation in the studies, which, with other documents attesting to their behavior in prison, would be reviewed by the Parole Board. Studies had been undertaken with 4,000 volunteers on the Malaria Project during the last 20 years, and members of the Parole Board reviewed our letters with that perspective in mind. Finally, after they read it and we read it to them, the inmates signed a document with witnesses, which confirmed they were giving their informed consent to volunteer to take malaria, undertaken in accordance with the rules for medical studies, delineated in the Nuremberg Code and in the Helsinki Declaration—rules for the proper conduct of studies involving human subjects.

THE NUREMBERG CODE

1. The voluntary consent of the human subject is absolutely essential.
2. The experiment should be such to yield fruitful results for the good of society, unprocurable by other methods or means of study, and not random and unnecessary in nature.
3. The experiment should be so designed and based on the results of animal experimentation and a knowledge of the natural history of the disease or other problem under study that the anticipated results will justify the performance of the experiment.
4. The experiment should be conducted as to avoid all unnecessary physical and mental suffering and injury.
5. No experiment should be conducted where there is an a priori reason to believe that death or disabling injury will occur, except, perhaps, in those experiments where the experimental physicians also serve as subjects.
6. The degree of risk to be taken should never

exceed that determined by the humanitarian importance of the problem to be solved by the experiment.

7. Proper preparations should be made and adequate facilities provided to protect the experimental subject against even remote possibilities of injury, disability, or death.

8. The experiment should be conducted only by scientifically qualified persons. The highest degree of skill and care should be required through all stages of the experiment of those who conduct or engage in the experiment.

9. During the course of the experiment the human subject should be at liberty to bring the experiment to an end if he has reached the physical or mental state where continuation of the experiment seems to him to be impossible.

10. During the course of the experiment the scientist in charge must be prepared to terminate the experiment at any stage, if he has probable cause to believe, in the exercise of good faith, superior skill and careful judgment required of him that a continuation of the experiment is likely to result in injury, disability, or death to the experimental subject.

Consent to Participate

After the volunteer read, discussed, and signed two copies of the document giving his consent to participate, witnesses affixed their signatures. One copy was filed in our office of the Malaria Project, the other was deposited at The University of Chicago.

This was the document our former volunteer, **Nathan F. Leopold**, requested in his letter addressed to the "Officer-in-Charge, Malaria Project, Illinois State Penitentiary," dated 8 February 1965. He asked for a blank copy of this "release" (consent to participate) to use in studies with drugs to treat intestinal parasitism in volunteer inmates in a prison in Puerto Rico while he served as a research associate in the Social Service Program of the Puerto Rican Department of Public Health. He had signed such a document in 1945 when he had volunteered to take malaria on the Malaria Project in Stateville.

Nathan Leopold was recognized for his research efforts by election to honorary membership in the American Society of Tropical Medicine & Hygiene in 1965, the same year I was elected to membership in that scientific society.

WHY VOLUNTEER?

"Why would an inmate volunteer for our malaria studies?" I asked Danny, our inmate clerk.

Danny replied with something like this, as I remember it, "Well, Doc, some of these men have brothers in the Army, and want to do some good for them and for society, but they probably would never admit it. Knowing many men have volunteered in the past without being injured, they know they will be well cared for, and some are proud to take risks the 'man-on-the-street' would be afraid to take, machismo."

"These guys are not under the illusion that your letter to the Parole Board, which has seen so many letters for men who volunteered to take malaria over the years, will get them early parole. Yes, they will receive a small stipend to spend in the Commissary, but it is a lot less than they could get donating blood, which they can never do if they take malaria. Another thing, being hospitalized for several weeks during the studies breaks the monotony of prison life and helps them 'do time'," Danny said.

Herpes Zoster, "Shingles"

One of the volunteers, we rejected, only because his urinary sediment contained a granular cast of questionable significance, was disappointed he was not chosen. So the inmate, Marlin, wrote a letter to the Catholic Chaplain asking him to appeal our decision. Attesting to Marlin's sincerity and the depth of his faith, Father Brinkman asked us if we would reconsider. Impressed with Marlin's commitment, we repeated the tests, found no abnormalities, and we agreed to permit him to participate in the studies of malaria.

During the first few days he had fever in the early stages of his malaria infection, I noticed redness in Marlin's left eye when I was making rounds. Occasionally, patients would get cold sores, *Herpes simplex* activation, on their lips with fevers. As (bad) luck would have it, Marlin's fever had activated dormant *Herpes zoster*, a viral herpetic eruption usually located on the trunk (zoster=Greek for girdle), but rarely, as in his case, on the cranial nerves of the head and neck; i.e., in the Ophthalmic branch of his left fifth cranial nerve. This had never happened before. I stopped the study immediately, cured his malaria with intravenous quinine, and I spent the next two days, with help from our staff, applying a new ophthalmic antiviral agent, Idoxuridine (IUDR) eye drops to his left eye every two hours to prevent blistering of the cornea. Thank goodness, the redness subsided, no blisters occurred, and he sustained no damage to his cornea.

Except for the *H. zoster* activation, which caused no damage to Marlin's eye, there were no untoward events in 300 inmates who volunteered to participate in studies of drug-resistant falciparum malaria from 1962 to 1964. Despite resistance to the many newer antimalarial drugs, we could suppress the parasites in the blood and cure all of the infections with the administration of intravenous quinine sulfate to volunteers infected with chloroquine-resistant strains of *Plasmodium falciparum* from Southeast Asia. The Army provided us with more than adequate supplies of quinine for our studies, but the drug was scarce, and we had to discover new regimens for preventing and curing this recalcitrant malaria. With the commitment of our volunteers, and the efforts of our staff, we did.

Professor Alf S. Alving, MD, Director

Invariably, Dr. Alving visited us at Stateville every Friday afternoon to review our study designs, results, and manuscripts. Either Robin or I had seen Dr. Alving in his office at The University of Chicago Hospitals & Clinics on the Tuesday before, when we had attended our weekly clinic, Renal Vascular Clinic for Robin, Hematology Clinic for me. After finishing our work on the Malaria Project, Alf chatted with Shirley. Then he kidded our inmate staff, offering them contraband items, like empty cigar tins, but they laughed, went along with his gag, never falling for his silly game of trying to get them in trouble for breaking the rules.

After we took care of things on the wards late Friday afternoons, we left the Project for a social hour at the Powells' house. We worried about Alf's return trip to Chicago on the interstate, driving his little red Ford Falcon, so Julie Powell made supper for Alf on many occasions. One time, when he extracted his handkerchief from his trousers pocket, we saw that he had patched a hole in it with staples and adhesive tape. Julie cheerfully picked up needle and thread and repaired it properly.

Although Alf had some help in caring for Dorothy, his wife—now in a wheelchair afflicted with multiple sclerosis for the past 25 years—Alf did all the grocery shopping, prepared the meals, and nursed his wife, lifting her on to the toilet or into bed. Unlike some patients with multiple sclerosis who were euphoric, in her later years Dorothy became paranoid. Despite Alf's unstinting care, she once telephoned the police to tell them that he was plotting to kill her. Alf was able to find a surrogate caregiver to stay with Dorothy Friday afternoons, giving him a respite to visit us, which he enjoyed.

The Audit

In September 1963, after I had been on the job a little over a month, Robin and I hosted two auditors from the Federal Government, who arrived at Stateville with a long list of laboratory instruments and equipment for which they asked us to account. Their five-page record listed University of Chicago inventory numbers and inaccurate descriptions of items purchased over the last 20 years. Most of our instruments and equipment had the metallic adhesive tags with the university inventory number applied, but some did not. It took the University Business Office a while to issue inventory numbers after the purchase of a piece of equipment, so there was a lag time between the receipt of an instrument and the issue of the tag with the number on it. It turned out that one of Alf's secretaries, not relating an earlier purchase to a late arriving number, had thrown some of the tags in the back of her desk drawer or in the wastebasket in Chicago without dispatching them to Stateville.

The senior auditor, in his blue business suit, was especially abrasive, beginning with, "I don't mean to be rude, doctor, but…" then he was exactly that, implying that we had defrauded the government. Fortunately for me, Robin took full responsibility to identify every piece of equipment on the auditor's list, finding every single one, some of which were obsolete and stored on shelves in our locked storeroom, next to the insectary in the hospital basement. Thereafter, for 30 years of running a research laboratory, I kept my own inventory of items purchased on grants, never trusting the bureaucracy of the university to retain my records.

FRIDAY, 22 NOVEMBER 1963

"Doc! The President's been shot! Someone shot Kennedy!" our inmate nurse shouted as he rushed into our conference room and turned on the television set. Shirley, Robin, several inmate staff members, and I stood transfixed, watching as the TV news reporter described the pandemonium unfolding at Dealey Plaza in Dallas, Texas. As his motorcade passed the Texas Book Depository and the grassy knoll on Elm Street, **President John F. Kennedy** had been shot while riding in his open limousine at 12:30 pm on Friday, 22 November 1963. An hour later, we learned the President had died at 1:00 pm in the Emergency Room at Parkland Hospital where the Secret Service had raced his limousine after the shooting.

Later that afternoon, Dallas Police apprehended **Lee Harvey Oswald**, the alleged assassin. After Oswald, ex-Marine, defector to Russia, and Cuban sympathizer, was questioned in the Dallas Police Station, he was being transferred to the county jail. In the basement of the Police Station, during the transfer, in full view of the TV cameras, **Jack Ruby** stepped out from the crowd and shot Oswald in the abdomen with a 0.38 caliber revolver. Police recovered from shock, grabbed Ruby, and rushed Oswald to Parkland Hospital, where he died at 1:07 pm Sunday, 24 November 1963.

Released on 27 September 1964, the final report of the **Warren Commission**, appointed by President Lyndon B. Johnson and chaired by Chief Justice of the Supreme Court, Earl Warren, declared that President John F. Kennedy had been killed by a lone assassin, a Marxist, Lee Harvey Oswald, firing an Italian Mannlicher-Carcano

Army Carbine from a sixth floor window of the Texas Book Depository in Dallas, Texas, on 22 November 1963.

ULTIMATE SACRIFICE

What really happened, and why has it taken over half a century for the truth to come out? In a nutshell, the murder was a Mafia hit, covered up by organized crime lords, the CIA, Attorney General Robert F. Kennedy, and the Press. Documentation to support this opinion can be found in Waldron, Lamar & Hartmann, Thom: *Ultimate Sacrifice-John and Robert Kennedy, the Plan for a Coup in Cuba, and the Murder of JFK,* Carroll & Graf Publishers, New York, 2005, pp. 904. Seventeen years in preparation, this book contains reports of eye witnesses, information from the review of classified documents released under the Freedom of Information Act, from the US National Archives, the Joint Chiefs of Staff, the CIA, the FBI, and from other sources, including the files of the Soviet KGB.[¶]

Tuesdays

Every other Tuesday afternoon I attended the Hematology Clinic at The University of Chicago Hospitals & Clinics while Robin worked

---

[¶] Other authors reported evidence of the Mafia hit, unavailable to the members of the Warren Commission, that contradicted the conclusions in the Warren Commission Report: Giancana, Sam & Giancana, Chuck: *Double Cross,* Warner Books, New York, NY, 1992, pp. 366; Hersh, Seymour M.: *The Dark Side of Camelot,* Little, Brown & Co., Boston, 1997, pp. 498; Talbot, David: *Brothers, The Hidden History of the Kennedy Years,* Free Press, New York, NY, 2007, pp. 478; Childs, MD, Allen: *We Were There; Revelations from the Dallas Doctors Who Attended to JFK on November 22, 1963,* Skyhorse Publishing, New York, NY, 2013, pp. 167; Vaccara, Stefano: *Carlos Marcello, The Man Behind the JFK Assassination,* Enigma Books, New York, NY, 2015, pp. 200.

at Stateville, taking call on the Malaria Project that night. I covered for him on alternate Tuesdays when he attended the Renal Vascular Section's Nephrology Clinic.

The Army had finally replaced our 1960 Ford Sedan, a piece of junk, with a brand new 1964 Chevrolet Station Wagon. On Tuesday morning, after filling the tank with gasoline at the Texaco Station in Plainfield, I drove northeast at 70 miles per hour to Chicago on historic Route 66, popularized by singer Nat King Cole: "Get your kicks on Route 66," now improved as Interstate 55. Some Tuesdays, as I was leaving Plainfield, I saw George Block fueling his new baby-blue Cadillac convertible at the Texaco Station. Halfway to Chicago on I-55, I heard a familiar auto horn behind me. I would look in vain for George in my rear view mirror, return my gaze forward, and see him pulling away in front of me, waving as he passed me doing at least 85 miles per hour.

GEORGE BLOCK, MD, SURGEON

Dr. George Block was in his late 30's, 5'8" tall, stocky muscular frame, square asymmetric face (indented left forehead with scar over left eye), thinning, short prematurely gray hair, would impress a stranger as an ex-fighter. I met him in my last year as a Fellow in Hematology when he responded to our request for consultation for a patient with acute leukemia requiring surgery. The patient's low white blood cell and platelet counts discouraged other surgeons, faced with such risks, from operating. George operated in these desperate straits and pulled our patient through for a full recovery. We relied on him as a superb surgeon for our very ill patients.

Despite his appearance and unconventional attitude for a University of Chicago professor, George was a brilliant teacher of clinical medicine. He worked very hard, yet never had to work a day in his life. His family had owned Blockson Chemical Company in Joliet, Illinois, later sold to corporate giant, Olin-Matheson. His uncle, Leigh Block, benefactor of The University of Chicago and The Chicago Institute of Art, was President of Inland Steel Company.

A rarity on most college campuses, George Block must have been one of the few Republicans on the faculty of The University of Chicago. Several months after Lyndon Johnson won the Presidential Election of 1964, George remarked, "My Democrat friends told me if I voted for Senator Barry Goldwater instead of Johnson, there would be war in Vietnam and rioting in the streets of America. Well, I did, and there was."

On 8January1964, President Lyndon B. Johnson declared "War on Poverty." Until he served in public office, he was a Texas school teacher of modest means, but he enriched himself, winning his personal war on poverty, retiring from the Presidency in 1969, a wealthy man, to his ranch on the Pedernales River in the Texas Hill Country.

Hematology Clinic

One of the black patients in my Tuesday Hematology Clinic at The University of Chicago, Jane (not her real name), fought her war on poverty and changed my preconceived notion about ADC (Aid to Dependent Children) that encouraged black single mothers on Chicago's Southside to have babies.

Before Jane became pregnant, at age 17 years, her hemoglobin and red blood cells were lower than normal, because she had sickle cell anemia. Numerous painful crises requiring hospitalizations for hydration and pain relief interrupted her regular attendance at high school. As gestation progressed, her fetus consumed increasing amounts of her body's stores of folic acid, depriving her bone marrow of a metabolite essential to accommodate the accelerated red blood cell production necessary to compensate for their increased destruction, caused by the sickle cell disease. Her older sister, Jasmine (not her real name), when she was pregnant, and who also had sickle cell disease, suffered an aplastic crisis with extreme anemia and nearly died until transfused with blood and given supplemental folic acid. So I was alerted to Jane's needs and treated her appropriately.

Despite the high mortality for mother and fetus with sickle cell disease, both Jane and Jasmine survived to nurse healthy babies. Over the next two years, I learned that not only Jane and Jasmine had graduated from high school, but that their single mother had completed high school courses to receive her degree (GED), and now all three single mothers were gainfully employed.

The Trip Home

While I attended Hematology Clinic on Tuesday afternoons, Dr. Alving's laboratory assistants packed the supplies in the Army Station Wagon that Robin, Shirley, and I had ordered for the Malaria Project. Driving southwest out of Chicago for Plainfield during winter months, I found that the slushy ice-covered I-55/US-66 on dark Tuesday nights was challenging, to say the least. Our new Chevy Station Wagon, which performed so well on dry pavement, tended to "fish-tail" (rear wheels slid sideways) on slippery surfaces, forcing me to cut the speed to 37 miles per hour. Semi-trailer trucks roared by in the dark at 70 mph, spraying my windshield with slush and dirt, so that I could barely see the road.

Adding to my anxiety, were sounds coming from the supplies in back of the station wagon, sounds of inflammable and corrosive liquids, acetone and sulfuric acid, sloshing around in 5-gallon drums. Heaving a sigh of relief, I arrived home without incident to reflect that I had been driving a "car bomb" down the expressway that night.

Following my Tuesday trip to the University of Chicago, I picked up Robin at his house on Wednesday morning in the Army Station Wagon and drove us to work. At the entrance to the Administration Building, I watched two inmates unload our supplies from the station wagon to a cart. Robin returned the station wagon to the parking lot. An inmate pushed our cart holding our supplies, and we proceeded to the hospital elevator. Shortly after greeting Shirley, I relaxed in the notion that none of our supplies, including drugs and chemicals, had left my sight until she locked them securely in the Malaria Project Pharmacy/Nursing Station.

It was probably after the second time that I brought the supplies from Chicago to Stateville that Robin and I responded to an urgent summons to appear at Warden Pate's Office. Sitting next to Warden Pate was the Prison Pharmacist, scowling with an accusatory look on his face. Holding a copy of our list of supplies, which we always gave the Pharmacist, Warden Pate said, "Doc, the Pharmacist pointed out that one of the items you brought in today was a jar of **Sodium Cyanide**. What if an inmate got hold of some of that and laced it on the food served to us in Staff Dining Room downstairs?"

We responded with a detailed review of all of our security procedures, including the fact that sodium cyanide had been used in our assays of erythrocyte glutathione over the past ten years, and this was the first time that the Prison Pharmacist happened to notice it on our list of supplies, provided to him each time a jar of the chemical was brought into the Project over those many years. Our explanation seemed to satisfy Warden Pate, and we renewed our vigilance regarding the disposition of the drugs and chemicals for which we were responsible.

Our Fallen Chief

In April 1964, shortly after we returned from a weekend in St. Louis, Robin called me to say that, Dr. Alving had become depressed and slit his throat and wrists with a kitchen knife. He had survived his attempted suicide, because Isabel, his secretary, worried, because he was late to arrive at his office in the hospital, went to his home to find him unresponsive on the kitchen floor in a pool of blood. Recovering from her shock, she called an ambulance. Physicians transfused blood, saving his life, but the blood loss from the self-inflicted wounds had led to hemorrhagic shock and a stroke, leaving him with hemiplegia and loss of speech, from which he never recovered.

Would Dr. Alving's inability to direct the University of Chicago-Army Medical Research Project, which he had so ably managed for 20 years, mean the end of it? Completing our mission to discover the prevention and treatment for multi-drug resistant falciparum malaria depended upon the decisions of leaders in three large institutions, our inmate volunteers, our staff, and our selves. Uncertainty and anxiety about the decisions those responsible for our fate might make arose from knowing that Alf's management style was to "play his cards close to his chest," i.e., he rarely revealed to us the consultations he had had with his superiors.

Alf's boss was, **Leon O. Jacobson, MD**, Chairman of Medicine, at The University of Chicago. Jake assured Robin and me that the University would continue to sponsor the Malaria Project if the Surgeon General of the Army and the Warden at Stateville agreed it should continue.

Robin telephoned **Brigadier General Robert E. Blount**, the Surgeon General in Washington. Dr. Blount liked Alf and expressed his heartfelt condolences. He said that he, and the officers in the

Army Medical Corps, regarded our research mission vital to the health of our troops in Southeast Asia. General Blount assured us that the Army would continue to support the Malaria Project, pending approval by the Warden at Stateville.

An inmate orderly in blue denims showed Robin and me into a comfortably furnished sitting room in the home of **Warden Frank Pate**. He lived with his wife and teenage daughter in a house just outside the wall on the grounds of the penitentiary. Having known Dr. Alving for 20 years, his expression was one of sorrow and thoughtful concern as he listened to Robin relate the circumstances that had led us to this sad late afternoon visit. At the end of Robin's narrative, Warden Pate expressed his sympathy for Alf's condition and for our uncertainty, and said, "Of course the Malaria Project will have our continued support at Stateville. It's part of us here."

Without being summoned, the inmate orderly appeared at the door with a tray carrying three glasses with ice cubes and set it on the coffee table in front of us. Warden Pate turned and reached into a cabinet from which he extracted a bottle of Scotch and poured each of us an ounce of the golden liquid. We imbibed, relaxed, and recalled anecdotes of good times with Dr. Alving and discussed our plans for the Project.

ALF SVEN ALVING, MD (8 MARCH 1902-18 MAY 1965)

Neighbors knocked on the door of the Alving home in Iron Mountain, Michigan, asking to see the Alvings' son, "the ugliest baby in town," said **Rhoda Estrem** (not her real name), as she sat talking to me in an examining room of my Tuesday afternoon Hematology Clinic. She was a former patient of Dr. Alving who had been referred to my care after his stroke.

A plump woman in her early 70's, she supplemented her Social Security income by writing children's stories for publications displayed at grocery store check-out counters.

A retired nurse, Miss Estrem had known Alf since he arrived with his mother from Sweden to live in Rhoda's hometown of Iron Mountain, Michigan, in the state's Upper Peninsula. Alf loved to tell his straightlaced colleagues he was illegitimate, having been carried by his mother as a baby while she pursued his father as he chased his mistress to America. Alf's father may have married his mother, because Alf's Curriculum *Vitae*, dated September 1963 states:

> "Born: March 8, 1902 (Sweden) Derivative U.S.
> Citizenship by Father's Naturalization, 1920"

Miss Estrem said Alf's father was known as an excellent general practitioner whose reputation extended beyond Iron Mountain. She told me of a patient from there who sought care at the esteemed Mayo Clinic in Rochester, Minnesota. After his examination, the patient said the Mayo Physician asked him, "Why would you come here to see us when the **'Swedish Jesus'** (Dr. Alving) practices in your town?"

Iron Mountain, Michigan, on Wisconsin's northeast border, with a population of about 8,000 persons, may have been slightly more remote than Cheboygan, my father's hometown on the northern tip of mainland Michigan. Born six months after my father, Alf left for college in Ann Arbor a couple of years after my dad arrived there. They were contemporaries at The University of Michigan, but I never heard my father say he knew Alf as a college student then. My father graduated from Medical School there in 1928 and left for an internship at Cleveland City Hospital that year.

Alf attained his BS in 1925, and his MD in 1927, followed by internship and residency at the University of Michigan Hospital,

1927-1929. From 1929-1934, he served as Assistant Resident Physician at the **Rockefeller Institute for Medical Research**, where he worked five years in the laboratory of the renowned expert on kidney physiology, Dr. Donald Van Slyke.

In 1934, Dr. Alving joined the faculty of The University of Chicago as Chief, Section of Renal Vascular Disease, Department of Medicine, and Attending Physician, Albert Merritt Billings Hospital. During World War II, he was promoted to Full Professor of Medicine in 1944, when he was also named Principal Investigator (Director) of the University of Chicago-Army Medical Research Project, Stateville Penitentiary, Joliet, Illinois.

ALF'S HUMOR

Alf was devoted to his family, yearning for times happier than he experienced in his childhood, but his emotional strength was sorely tested in the years before his death. Dorothy, his wife, had become progressively disabled with multiple sclerosis over the last 25 years; their eldest son, as a young man, had been diagnosed with glomerulonephritis and severe hypertension (Alf's medical specialty); and his mother, in her 80's, had leukemia. Other disappointments may have led to Alf's acerbic, sarcastic, dark sense of humor. He once introduced me to one of his young adult sons as, "my idiot child." His son didn't like that much. Neither did I.

Charley Pak, a brilliant, modest medical student of Korean ethnicity, worked in Alf's laboratory during his elective course in research and later became a distinguished Professor of Medicine at Southwestern Medical School in Dallas, Texas. He earned an international reputation for his research on kidney stone formation, an expert in the field. His son earned the top score on the college SAT examination. One day, Alf walked into his lab and said, "Charley, I am surrounded by so many idiots that I don't know how to classify them. Except for you, Charley, you're a Mongolian Idiot."

In a small utility closet next to his office, Alf kept a photo-copier, a mimeograph machine, and an early version of a Xerox machine, to replicate the dozens of reports required by the bureaucracies of the Army, the University, and the State of Illinois, related to the Malaria Project. He called it his "Institute of Asexual Reproduction." In the presence of a patient he had just examined in the clinic, he called me, then a resident assigned to his service, to come into the examining room and do the "Whing—Ding," he meant the pelvic examination. An Alvingism, remembered by Alf's academic colleagues was, "The three most overrated things in the world were: *chicken-a-la-king*, sexual intercourse, and the Johns Hopkins Hospital." Some of Alf's wit drew honest laughter, but other remarks were so inappropriate or insulting, his listeners laughed out of embarrassment.

Finally, after months of care in the Chicago Institute of Rehabilitation, with little obvious improvement in his speech or paralysis, Alf was transferred to a nursing home in the Beverly Hills neighborhood of Chicago where Dorothy was receiving care after his stroke left him unable to provide her care.

Alf died 18 May 1965 at the age of 63 of "chronic essential hypertension and chronic cardiovascular disease," or of a broken heart. My friend and colleague, Jim Bowman, MD, who knew Alf well, attended a Commemoration Service for Dr. Alving at 8:00 pm, Monday, 7 June 1965, at Bethany Union Church in Chicago. Karen and I joined this church after my military service when I became a member of the faculty at The University of Chicago. Jim Bowman and I sat in a pew at the back of this dimly lit hushed church. As the first chords of the opening hymn were struck on the organ, a bat flew from behind the altar, down the aisle, over our heads, and out the open door in the back. Jim and I turned to each other and said in unison, "My God, it's Alf!"

JAKE'S TRIBUTE

Alf, Jake, and my father were members of the Association of American Physicians, as were most Nobel Laureates in Medicine. After Alf died, his boss, Leon O. "Jake" Jacobson, MD, Chairman, Department of Medicine, published a tribute to him in the prestigious *Transactions of the Association of American Physicians*, v. lxxix, p. 16, 1966; Alf Sven Alving 1902-1965, from which I quote in part:

> "...His (Alf's) contributions to our understanding of the kidney, hypertension, and renal disease are alone sufficient to place him high in the ranks of distinguished investigators and clinicians."
>
> "...A virtually new career in another capacity began for Alving during World War II when he was literally drafted into the field of chemotherapy of malaria and set up the malaria project at Stateville Penitentiary. This project, soley through the efforts of Alving and his chosen associates, has represented a union of the highest order between so-called theoretical and applied research with results that have been of tremendous significance in both respects. The early contributions were devoted to the more straight-forward aspects of the problem, which developed over the years into a remarkable program in chemotherapy ranging from studies of compounds under field conditions to fundamental investigations into the mechanism of drug toxicity. These, in turn, led to the discovery of glucose-6-phosphate dehydrogenase deficiency."
>
> "...Alf Alving was a man of profound intellect who dearly loved to be underestimated. He was a jovial fellow with a magnificent earthy sense of

humor and a sharp wit that he often used to prick
any bubble of pretense or self-pity in the young
men associated with him or for that matter in his
colleagues on committees or at faculty meetings.
His almost fanatic devotion to his family was
well known. His intimate friends recognized and
cherished the fundamental sympathy and kindness
that underlay all his relationships with them. It
is hard to become reconciled to his loss. Leon O.
Jacobson."

SPRING 1964

The loss of Alf as Director of the Project was devastating, but we
struggled to recover the focus of our work. With the approval of the
leaders of the three institutions involved, The University of Chicago,
the U.S. Army, and Stateville Penitentiary—Robin D. Powell, MD,
and Paul E. Carson, MD, were named co-directors of the University
of Chicago-Army Medical Research Project. Both Robin and Paul
had their primary appointments in the Department of Medicine
at The University of Chicago. Robin would soon complete his two
years of active duty with the Army, and a search for his successor had
begun. Karen and I anticipated the arrival in July 1964 of his replacement, unknown that spring, but we were optimistic about what the
future might bring.

Part III. Stateville
(1964-1965)

Prologue

A sweet little girl standing in a sunny meadow appeared on the television screen. With hesitation she plucked the petals from a daisy, counting softly, "one, two, three, four,..." As her dulcet speech faded, a man's gruff voice took over the countdown for a ballistic missile launch. On the count of "10," the startled little girl looked up into the sky, where the television screen lit up with the horrific explosion of an atomic bomb. With the bomb's expanding mushroom cloud as background, the voice of President Lyndon Johnson warned, "These are the stakes—to make a world in which all God's children can live, or go into the dark. We must either love each other, or we must die." An announcer followed with, "Vote for President Johnson on November 3rd. The stakes are too high for you to stay home."

Shocking television viewers on 7 September 1964, members of the Democratic National Committee, who portrayed Johnson's Republican opponent, Senator Barry Goldwater, as a warmonger, played only once the "Daisy Ad," confident the liberal news media would replay it over and over again during the presidential election campaign of 1964. The TV "news" obliged. Johnson won his election of 1964 in a landslide.

Johnson called on Congress to pass the Gulf of Tonkin Resolution in August, essentially a declaration of war against North Vietnam, but he was quoted as saying, "None of our American boys in uniform will die on Asian soil." Yet, in September 1964, we medical officers at the Army Medical Research Project were told our Commander-in-Chief would deploy U.S. Combat Troops to the malarious regions of Vietnam after the election in November 1964. As a consequence, we were directed to accelerate our search for drugs to prevent and cure chloroquine-resistant falciparum malaria, which was prevalent there.

For 15 years, chloroquine had served throughout the world as the mainstay drug to prevent and treat infections with falciparum malaria. By 1964, however, strains of *Plasmodium falciparum* from Southeast Asia, and from South America, had proved resistant not only to chloroquine, but also to other previously effective anti-malarial drugs, like hydroxychloroquine, amodiaquine, atabrine (mepacrine, quinacrine) pyrimethamine, paludrine, and to newer experimental drugs like cycloguanil pamoate (CI-501), and 377C54 (an hydoroxynaphthalene derivative).

Approval of new drugs by the Federal Drug Administration (FDA) took years, and we were given but several months to come up with prophylactic and therapeutic regimens effective against multi-drug resistant falciparum malaria that would protect our troops from this potentially lethal disease. So, our mission was clear, but the path to solving this problem was not. Its solution required thought, review of the scientific literature, more thought, and then a research effort dependent upon a commitment by volunteers, staff, and good fortune.

Eureka!

DDS

Two of the four men who volunteered to receive the bites of *Anopheles stephensi* mosquitoes infected with multi-drug resistant Malayan

(Camp) Strain of *Plasmodium falciparum* never came down with malaria; no symptoms, and no parasites on repeated thick smears of their blood. Both had been taking a small daily oral dose of Dapsone (4,4'-diaminodiphenyl sulfone or DDS). One of them had also received a small daily dose of pyrimethamine with the DDS. Of the two other volunteers in the "bite group" of four, both developed symptoms of malaria and blood containing parasites on thick smears. One man had taken pyrimethamine alone, and the other had taken no medication. The intravenous administration of quinine sulfate cured both volunteers of malaria.

PREVENTION

Robin, Ben and I reviewed these results, suppressed, "Wow!" and wondered aloud if DDS was the answer to the problem we hoped to solve. Well, it was, and it wasn't. Although later studies showed DDS had a suppressive effect on an acute attack of drug-resistant falciparum malaria, it acted slowly and failed to induce a radical cure. But the good news was that it prevented mosquito-induced malaria in volunteers taking a relatively small dose of DDS.**

Results of extensive subsequent studies led to a meeting of military leaders, scientists from the National Institutes of Health, and others in May 1965 at the University of Chicago-Army Medical Research Project in our conference room in Stateville Penitentiary. After review of our findings and deliberation, our commanding officer authorized the initiation of field trials of DDS in Vietnam to determine if it would protect our troops exposed to drug-resistant malaria. Before universal application of our preventive regimen could be introduced,

** DeGowin, Richard L., Eppes, R. Bennett, Carson, Paul E., and Powell, Robin D.: "The Effects of Diaphenylsulfone (DDS) against Chloroquine-resistant," *Plasmodium falciparum*, Bulletin World Health Organization, *34*:671-681, 1966.

more soldiers were evacuated from Vietnam with malaria in 1965 than those sent home with battle wounds. Later, when our DDS regimen was broadly issued, it proved to be an effective preventive measure. Our volunteers took justifiable pride in their service, which received positive notice in the local, national, and international press.

SULFONES

I recognized his name as senior author of a scientific paper written before World War II, evaluating the efficacy of Promin as an anti-malarial drug.[††] As Dean of The University of Chicago School of Medicine, **Lowell T. Coggeshall, MD** signed my diploma, Doctor of Medicine, dated 12 June 1959.

Sulfones like promin were set aside in the 1940's as therapeutic agents, because atabrine seemed to be a better prophylactic against malaria, and before the discovery of penicillin, sulfonamides appeared less toxic than sulfones in the treatment of bacterial infections.

A fascinating series of events occurred in the 30-some years following the synthesis of sulfones and sulfonamides by the I.G. Farbenindustrie, the German dye manufacturer. The parent sulfone, DDS, was absorbed well taken orally, and it had substantial anti-bacterial activity, but it was 20 times more toxic than a sulfonamide when administered in equivalent dosage. So, to mitigate its toxicity, chemists synthesized compounds like promin (glucosulfone) by add-ing side-chains to DDS, requiring intravenous administration. But later metabolic studies revealed that the body cleaved the side-chains from the parent compound, leaving DDS as the active chemical

---

[††] Coggeshall, L.T., Maier, J. and Best, C.A.: The Effectiveness of Two New Types of Chemotherapeutic Agents in Malaria: Sodium P,P'-Diaminondiphenylsulfone, N,N' Didextrose-sulfonate (Promin) and 2-Sulfanilamido Pyrimidine (Sulfadia-zine), JAMA 117:1077-1081, 1941.

moiety. Administering conjugated molecules, like promin, simply reduced the dose of DDS.

Indeed, veterinarians discovered if they administered DDS in a dosage lower than they would ordinarily prescribe a sulfonamide for treating streptococcal mastitis in dairy cows, the sulfone was effective and less toxic than feared.

Leprosy

In another sphere, physician scientists discovered sulfones exhibited activity against *Mycobacterium tuberculosis* and *Mycobacterium leprae*. Streptomycin supplanted sulfones in the treatment of tuberculosis, but small doses of sulfones proved effective in controlling leprosy. Interestingly, leprologists treating their patients with sulfones, cared for in leper colonies located in regions of endemic malaria, reported their patients did not come down with malaria. Moreover, a daily dose of 50 mg of DDS was sufficient to control a patient's leprosy and prevent them from contracting malaria.

My teachers and friends, dermatologists Drs. Al Lorincz, Fred Malkinson, and Roger Pearson, suggested that sulfones acted on the tissues inflamed by leprosy. They used DDS with good response treating chronic inflammatory skin diseases, like dermatitis herpetiformis, and pyoderma gangrenosa. Good responses, however, required daily doses of DDS exceeding 500-1000 mg, which caused transient anemia and a reactive reticulocytosis.

Can you teach an old dog new tricks?

A review of the literature concerning DDS, and the realization that leprologists and dermatologists were using DDS in their daily practice, led me to design, with Robin's help, the clinical studies that proved fruitful.

The Army was faced with an urgent need to issue medication to their troops in Vietnam to prevent infections by multi-drug resistant falciparum malaria. Recognizing the fact that clinicians had been prescribing DDS for over 30 years meant that we were not recommending the use of a "new drug," requiring extensive testing in laboratory animals and clinical trials. Accepting a "new drug" for the use by the Army might take months and years of testing and reviews by committees to obtain approval by the Federal Drug Administration, an agency hypersensitive to possible side-effects of drugs available to the public, because of the congenital defects (phocomelia) encountered with the use of Thalidomide in Europe.

R. Bennett Eppes, MD

When it became clear that Dr. Alving would not recover enough from his stroke to direct the University of Chicago-Army Medical Research Project, my partner, Robin Powell, was named Clinical Director, and Paul Carson was named Scientific Director of the Malaria Project. As co-directors, they started searching for Robin's replacement, my new partner, anticipating Robin's discharge from two year's active duty in the U.S. Army Medical Corps, his separation expected in early July 1964. But they had difficulty finding a medical officer who wanted to spend two years of his life in a maximum security prison.

Uncertainty and anxiety until the eleventh hour, yielded a pleasant surprise when Robin and Paul, with recruit in tow, walked into our Conference Room on the 3rd floor of the Stateville Prison Hospital on a warm morning late in July 1964. Perspiring in his khaki uniform, the newcomer's eyes, wide open, shifted rapidly to the barred windows, to the inmates across the hall, and then to me. He said, "Hi. I'm Ben Eppes," and grasped my hand in a quick handshake, moist more from anxiety than humidity, lost eye contact, continued to assess the surroundings, wondering what he had volunteered for, wondering if he had made the right decision. He looked frightened.

We were fortunate Ben chose to serve on the Malaria Project for the next two years, 1964-1966. Captain R. Bennett Eppes, MC, USAR, was an excellent physician, intelligent, well-trained, and hard working. He graduated with an A.B. from Yale in 1958, received his M.D. in 1962 from the University of Pennsylvania, and completed a year of internship and a year as Resident in Internal Medicine at the University Hospitals of Western Reserve University in Cleveland, Ohio, before entering active duty in the Army Medical Corps with assignment to Walter Reed Army Institute of Research (WRAIR). After completing his service on active duty, he intended to become a Resident in Dermatology, returning to Western Reserve, which he did in 1966.

THE DOCTOR DRAFT

Some might consider the program discriminatory, but physicians had been deferred to finish their education before being drafted in the Army. During the Korean War (1950-1953), doctors were drafted until age 52, but by the 1960's the draft age had been lowered to 36. As the war in Vietnam heated up, the Doctor Draft touched many of my friends and colleagues, who volunteered for service to have some say in their assignments.

If I knew, I've forgotten the details of why Ben Eppes made the decision to request assignment to the Malaria Project. I surmise that he must have talked about the Project to Robert W. Kellermeyer, MD, Professor of Medicine and Hematology at Western Reserve University. Bob had preceded us in the late 1950's as an officer in the U.S. Public Health Service, assigned to the Malaria Project. He had made significant research contributions to our understanding of

Primaquine-sensitive hemolytic anemia while assigned to Stateville for his military service, and he had kept in contact with Paul Carson at The University of Chicago after his discharge from active duty. Then I learned that Ben's uncle, whom he must have asked about the Project, was William (Bill) Bennett Bean, MD, Professor and Head, Department of Internal Medicine, The University of Iowa, my father's boss, and an acquaintance of Dr. Alving.

THOMAS JEFFERSON, THE EPPES, AND THE HEMINGS

Ben Eppes's mother was Bill Bean's sister. Bill, excessively proud of his Virginia heritage, reminded me, as if I should have known, that Ben was descended from the Virginia Eppes, who were among the first colonists to arrive from England. Francis Eppes, the founding settler, served on the Council of Virginia in the 1630's. His descendant, Martha Eppes, daughter of Francis Eppes IV, married John Wayles in 1746 and brought mulatto slave Elizabeth Hemings as her property to her new home, *The Forest*. Martha Eppes died in 1748 after the birth of her daughter, Martha Wayles, leaving the Hemings slaves to her husband, John Wayles.

After his second and third white wives died, John Wayles took Elizabeth Hemings as his "concubine" with whom he had six children. Wayles last daughter, Sarah (Sally) Hemings (1773-1835), was born the year he died, and she became a house slave of white daughter Martha Wayles. Martha Wayles married Bathurst Skelton, who died within a year. Then, as a wealthy young widow, Martha Wayles Skelton married Thomas Jefferson in 1772. After Martha Wayles Skelton Jefferson died, Thomas Jefferson took Sally Hemings, his late wife's half-sister and slave, as his "concubine," who bore him seven children.

Maria (1778-1804), Thomas Jefferson's youngest white daughter and the granddaughter of Martha Eppes Wayles, married her cousin,

John Wayles Eppes in 1797. These relationships between the Eppes, Thomas Jefferson, and Hemings are documented in a work that received the National Book Award for 2008.[‡‡]

Times Change

When Robin became Co-Director of the Malaria Project, Julie and he built a house in Hinsdale, Illinois, conveniently located to O'Hare International Airport to the north, The University of Chicago to the east, and Stateville to the south. Robin planned his future with care, never leaving anything to chance. Cindy and Ben Eppes, with their infant daughter, and exuberant Kerry Blue Terrier, moved into the rental house in Plainfield where Robin and Julie had lived and had hosted us for many good times over the last year. Karen and I welcomed the Eppes. We invited them to our home during 1964-1965, but they had little interest in reciprocating, so I saw Ben every day at work, but rarely did we see his family.

Primaquine Sensitivity

Work by my predecessors on the Project showed that the 10% of African-American males with Primaquine-sensitive anemia (glucose-6-phosphate dehydrogenase deficiency) sustained a hemolytic anemia with a number of drugs other than Primaquine, including sulfonamides and sulfones.[§§]

My teacher and friend, hematologist **Dr. Ernest Beutler**, left the faculty of The University of Chicago to take jobs as Chairman of Medicine at City of Hope, and later, as Head of Research at Scripps

---

‡‡ Gordon-Reed, Annette: *The Hemingses of Monticello—An American Family*, W.W. Norton & Co., Inc., New York, pp. 798, 2008.
§§ Dern, R.J., Beutler, E., & Alving, A.S.: The Hemolytic Effect of PrimaquineV.,Primaquine Sensitivity as a Manifestation of a Multiple Drug Sensitivity, J. Lab. Clin. Med. 45: 30-39. 1955.

Medical Center in California. He first demonstrated decreased levels of reduced glutathione in G-6-PD deficient red blood cells, and later discovered the abnormal metabolism in several different blood diseases. His scholarship was recognized by election to the National Academy of Sciences. The *Los Angeles Times*, and the *New York Times*, reported that Ernie died 5 October 2008 at age 80 years of lymphoma.

To return, if we recommended issuing the drug as anti-malarial prophylaxis to thousands of combat troops, I needed to know if DDS caused anemia in healthy men, how severe it was in men with G-6-PD deficiency, and whether a daily dose of DDS that prevented acquisition of drug-resistant falciparum malaria caused significant hemolysis. I searched the scientific literature to find very little information about the severity of the hemolysis caused by DDS. The few papers I found reported observations of hemolysis in persons who were ill.

DDS for Treatment of Skin Disease

Dr. Alan Lorincz, Director of Dermatology, The University of Chicago, told me, in essence, "Daily doses of 500 to 1,000 mg DDS are required to treat patients afflicted with dermatitis herpetiformis or pyoderma gangrenosa. We see a mild anemia with a reactive reticulocytosis as we begin administering the drug, but red blood cell counts return to normal as we continue giving the medication."[5]

Anemia, Red Blood Cell Pathophysiology #101

An understanding of evolution informs us that mammals survive to reproduce if they replace blood lost from hemorrhage during childbirth, wounds, or injuries. During the summer of 1956, home in Iowa City, after completing my first year of medical school at

---

[5] Lorincz, A.L., & Pearson, R.W.: Sulfapyridine and Sulfone Type Drugs in Dermatology, Arch. Derm. 85:2-16, 1962.

The University of Chicago, I asked my father, a pioneer in Blood Banking, "How does a person's body replace the pint of blood he or she donates at your blood bank?" He said, "Leon Jacobson's research group at your medical school in Chicago is studying that very question." That question marked the beginning of my 30-year inquiry into the life and times of the erythrocyte, the red blood cell and its precursor, the hemopoietic stem cell.

The body's cells require oxygen to metabolize nutrients if they are to function and survive. Hemoglobin, the red pigment encased in red blood cells, binds oxygen from the inhaled atmosphere in the alveoli of the lungs and transports it to tissues at distant sites through blood vessels and capillaries, where it then releases it to the cells.

Blood is composed of cells (red and white blood cells and platelets) and fluid (plasma). When the concentration of red blood cells (RBC) falls below the normal range, measured in the laboratory by the RBC count, the hemoglobin concentration, and the hematocrit, the patient is said to have "anemia." But that just represents the beginning of understanding the problem. Discovering the mechanism of the anemia helps to identify its cause and to direct treatment of the patient's illness.

Normally, erythrocytes survive 120 days in the peripheral blood. This fact was discovered by Elmer DeGowin's research group using Ashby techniques, confirmed later by investigators observing the survival of 51Cr-labeled RBC. At the end of their life span, sustained by a progressively weakening carbohydrate metabolic energy producing system, RBC's are removed by macrophages in the spleen.

When the life span of the RBC is shortened by damage to the extent that its production by the bone marrow cannot compensate for the loss, *hemolysis* is said to be the mechanism of the anemia; a hemolytic anemia. Decreased concentration of RBC's (anemia) means that the oxygen-carrying capacity of the blood is diminished. This relative hypoxia (low oxygen) is sensed by an oxygen-binding heme protein in the renal (kidney) cortex that causes the release of the hormone erythropoietin, which circulates in the blood to induce the bone marrow to make more new RBC's, detected on special stains of blood smears as a reticulocytosis.

Perhaps the reader remembers the media reports of "red cell doping" in which erythropoietin, as *Epoietin*, was misused to increase the RBC concentration, the oxygen-carrying capacity of the blood, by bicyclers riding in the high altitude hypoxia of the mountains in the raceways of the Tour-de-France.

STUDIES OF DDS TOXICITY

Regarding the safe administration of DDS to our troops, while trying to prevent infections with multi-drug resistant falciparum malaria, why not simply add DDS to a test tube containing a suspension of RBC's in isotonic saline and determine at which concentration hemolysis occurred? I tried that with many variations, and it didn't work. It did not work, because the human body's metabolism was required for DDS to interact with protective mechanisms, damaging RBC's and making them vulnerable to removal from the circulation by macrophages in the spleen and liver.

Therefore, assessing the hemolytic toxicity of DDS to determine a safe dose depended upon inmates who would volunteer to participate in dose-response studies. When they learned of the proposed studies, inmates stepped forward and gave their informed consent to enter studies, conducted within the rules of the Nuremberg Code, in which they were exposed to maximum doses of DDS that were less than one-third of those currently prescribed by physicians treating patients with dermatitis herpetiformis, pyoderma gangrenosa, and other skin diseases.

Results of our studies showed, that unlike Primaquine, the larger daily doses of DDS (but smaller doses than used in treating patients with skin diseases) caused mild hemolysis in healthy volunteers. As expected from studies undertaken in the 1950's, such doses caused more hemolysis in healthy volunteers with G-6-PD deficiency than in those without the genetic defect. But to our relief, daily doses of DDS that protected volunteers against mosquito-induced infection with multi-drug resistant falciparum malaria, produced barely detectible, if any, shortening of the red blood cell life span. Moreover, none of the volunteers experienced symptoms or adverse side-effects while participating in these dose-response studies.***

Radical Cure with Pyrimethamine-Sulfadiazine

Following clues from experiments by other investigators, we discovered that a combination of drugs (Pyrimethamine/Sulfadiazine), commonly used to cure resistant toxoplasmosis, would cure, when taken orally, multi-drug resistant falciparum malaria. Nobel Laureate in Medicine (1988), **Dr. George H. Hitchings** called this technique using together a dihydrofolic reductase inhibitor (Pyrimethamine) and an inhibitor of paraminobenzoic acid (Sulfadiazine), a "sequential blockade of folate biosynthesis." Whereas, a malaria parasite might resist either drug singly, it could not replicate in the presence of both medicinal blocks to its metabolism. This finding meant that now we

---

*** DeGowin, R.L., Eppes, R.B., Powell, R.D. & Carson, P.E.: The Haemolytic Effects of Diaphenylsulfone (DDS) in Normal Subjects and in those with Glucose-6-phosphate dehydrogenase Deficiency, Bulletin World Health Organizaion, 35:165-179, 1966.

could recommend a regimen to elicit radical cure of drug-resistant malaria without relying on the use of intravenous quinine sulfate.[†††]

Bioethics

We were challenged to solve a significant problem. During World War II, 500,000 U.S. troops contracted malaria, 40,000 in the Korean War, with 300 deaths from malaria recorded in the two wars. Drugs effective to prevent more deaths then, didn't work now in Vietnam.

Certain clinical studies at Memorial-Sloan Kettering Hospital in the mid-1950's, and later at the Ohio State Penitentiary, engendered considerable debate in the scientific literature and lay press about how such studies should be undertaken.[‡‡‡]

During and since my service in the Army, I have thought a lot about the studies we undertook to discover a preventive regimen and radical cure of multi-drug resistant falciparum malaria. Not only did the results of our work benefit our troops sent by Presidents Kennedy and Johnson to help the people of South Vietnam defend themselves against oppression by the ruthless totalitarian government of North Vietnam, but we hoped that they stemmed the loss of millions of non-immune children dying of malaria every year in Africa and elsewhere.

By 1963, scientists throughout the world concluded *Plasmodium falciparum* parasites would not survive in tissue culture to permit testing of potential antimalarial drugs. Moreover, plasmodia that infected mice, *Plasmodium bergheii*, and those that infected other

[†††] Powell, R.D., DeGowin, R.L., & McNamara, J.V.: Clinical Experience with Sulfadiazine and Pyrimethamine in the treatment of Persons Experimentally Infected with Chloroquine-resistant Plasmodium falciparum, Ann. Tropical Medicine & Parasitology, 61:396-408, 1967

[‡‡‡] Science 143:551-553, 1964; Good Housekeeping 161:79,1965; JAMA 202:175-179, 1967.

non-human animals, responded differently to drugs than *P. falciparum* in humans, making the results of drug studies in animals with malaria unreliable predictors of efficacy and safety in patients.

I was reassured that physicians whom I respected had safely carried out antimalarial drug studies in over 4,000 inmates over the last 20 years without injury to the volunteers. Results of my predecessors' work on the Malaria Project at Stateville, showed us how to undertake studies safely to assess the efficacy and toxicity of antimalarial drugs in volunteers.

Undertaking such studies in the controlled conditions of a maximum security prison were critical to the safety of the inmate volunteers and the public. Radical cure of the study participant's malaria was mandatory before discharge from our hospital ward into the general prison population or his release from prison. So, the longer sentences of inmates incarcerated for murder and habitual criminality in Illinois's maximum security prison meant that a volunteer would not be released unexpectedly to the street with an active malarial infection.

Credit is due to **G. Robert Coatney, PhD** and **Peter G. Contacos, MD** of the National Institutes of Health, who conducted similar clinical studies of malaria in the Federal Penitentiary, Atlanta, Georgia.[§§§]

If you think about it, human beings are the only animals that "volunteer."

VOLUNTEERS
Learning from the experience of our predecessors, and from our own recent work, Ben, Shirley Hill, RN, our inmate nurses, and I were

---

[§§§] Contacos, P.G., Elder, H.A. & Coatney, G.R.: Therapeutic trials of a dihydroxynaphthalene (377C54) against *Plasmodium falciparum* and *Plasmodium vivax* infections in human volunteers; Am. J. Trop. Med. & Hyg. 12:513-518, 1963.

confident that we could at one time safely care for 8-12 volunteers participating in malaria studies. Since some of the regimens prevented attacks of acute malaria, less than the number of participating volunteers had fever or other symptoms in a study with two or three "bite groups" of four volunteers each.

Invariably, our notice of opening studies brought 14-18 inmates who applied to participate. Each was approved by the warden, and although they were healthy men between the ages of 20-40 years, with no illness detected by our history and physical examination, chest x-ray, blood counts, blood chemistries, and urinalysis, we asked six or more of the applicants to apply for subsequent studies. Our call for volunteers was always oversubscribed.

Ben, Shirley, Robin, and I met in our Conference Room with those inmates qualified to volunteer for a particular study, and we encouraged them to withdraw from participation if they had any reservations after listening to our detailed presentation of the benefits to society and the risks to them. We told them we strictly adhered to the dicta of the Nuremberg Code, rules for safely undertaking clinical research with volunteers. We said, "If you want to stop the study, we will stop it immediately and cure your malaria. If we think there is likelihood of injury, or for other reasons, we will stop the study." We gave each volunteer a written description of the study, detailing its risks and benefits, and a copy of the Nuremberg Code. Then we asked them to join us in signing two copies of the document before witnesses. One copy of the document was filed at Stateville, the other at The University of Chicago.

MOTIVES

Were inmates coerced to participate in studies of malaria? No. Most members of our inmate staff met us when they had volunteered to take malaria, participating in studies of antimalarial drugs. They had applied for jobs as nurses, clerks, and technicians on the Project after they had gotten to know us and we them. In their response to my question whether inmates were coerced to volunteer, they said something like this, "No, Doc. These guys think of this opportunity to volunteer as a privilege, even a right. They get time off from working in the Prison Factories, are hospitalized for several months, lie in bed, watch television, and several times a day are asked by you Docs and Nurse Hill how they are feeling. It's a change of scene. Many feel they are doing a 'good thing,' but probably wouldn't admit it."

Were the benefits of participating in our studies so great that they attracted men to volunteer from a sense of greed? I don't think so. The small stipend they received to spend in the Prison Commissary for volunteering was considerably less than they could be paid for donating blood to the blood banks. Of course, they were never permitted to donate blood if they had contracted malaria.

Our letter to the Parole Board recognizing an inmate's contribution to society as a volunteer on the Malaria Project was considered with the entire record of his behavior during his incarceration, but in later years the Board had received thousands of our letters, so the impact of our report was reviewed in that perspective. Early in the program, there was special recognition for volunteering to take malaria. On 19 June 1945, Nathan F. Leopold was one of the first 500 inmates to volunteer. As a result, Illinois Governor Adlai Stevenson commuted his 99-year sentence for kidnapping Bobby Franks on 21 May 1924 to 85 years, permitting Leopold to appear before the Parole Board in 1953. He was finally released in 1958, the year his autobiography, *Life Plus 99 Years*, was published.

THE DEDICATION

Inmates expressed their pride in participating in the studies of antimalarial drugs. The magazine *Joliet-Stateville Time,* published monthly by inmates in the Stateville Vocational School, distributed to inmates and staff in both institutions, described news about malaria research at Stateville in several issues. My copy of *Time*, April 1968, pp. 18-23, features the cover story: "Inmates Declare War on Mosquito," in which the history and current activities of the Malaria Project were reviewed in illustrated articles. One article reported the formal dedication and installation at Stateville by Warden Frank J. Pate and inmate volunteers, on 4 March 1968, of a bronze plaque in memory of Dr. Alving:

"In Memory of Alf Sven Alving, MD 1902-1965
Founder and Director 1944-1964 of
The University of Chicago-Army Medical
Research Project at Stateville Penitentiary."

A caption of a photograph of Warden Frank J. Pate, with prison physician Julius Venckus at his side, quoted Warden Pate (in part): "Dedication of this memorial plaque is small tribute to pay to a great doctor and scientist for his untiring efforts on behalf of humanity."

Guests attending the dedication of the plaque honoring Dr. Alving at Stateville included: Gustave J. Dammin, MD, President of the Armed Forces Epidemiology Board, Friedman Professor of Pathology at Harvard University, and Pathologist-in-Chief of Peter Bent Brigham Hospital in Boston; Leon O. Jacobson, MD, Dean of the Division of Biological Sciences and School of Medicine, The University of Chicago; David P. Earle, Jr., MD, Professor and Chairman, Department of Medicine, Northwestern University School of Medicine; and Hans H. Hecht, MD, Professor and Chairman, Department of Medicine, The University of Chicago.

Other friends and colleagues whom I recognize standing with me in the group photograph of the dedication are: Karl Reickmann, MD, James V. McNamara, MD, Paul E. Carson, MD, Robin D.

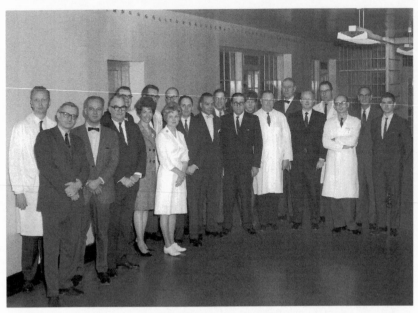

Guests attending the **Dedication of a Plaque** made by inmates in memory of **Alf Sven Alving, MD; Stateville, 4March1968.**

[Standing, left to right]

Karl Reickmann, MD, Malaria Project.

Hans H. Hecht, MD; Professor & Chairman, Department of Medicine, The University of Chicago.

Theodore N. Pullman, MD; Professor of Medicine, The University of Chicago.

David P. Earle, Jr., MD; Professor & Chairman, Department of Medicine, The Northwestern University School of Medicine.

Paul E. Carson, MD; Scientific Director, Malaria Project, Assistant Professor of Medicine, The University of Chicago.

Ann E. Lawrence, MD; Director of Endocrinology, Loyola University Medical School.

Thomas Stockert, MD; Malaria Project.

Shirley Hill, RN; Nurse Director, Malaria Project.

Richard L. DeGowin, MD; Assistant Professor of Medicine, The University of Chicago.

Alvin R. Tarlov, MD; Associate Professor of Medicine, The University of Chicago.

James E. Bowman, MD; Professor & Director, Clinical Pathology Laboratories, The University of Chicago Hospitals & Clinics.

Richard L. Landau, MD; Professor & Director, Endocrinology, The University of Chicago.

Frank J. Pate; Warden, Stateville Penitentiary, Joliet, Illinois. Unknown.

Julius Venckus, MD; Prison Physician, Stateville.

Gustave J. Dammin, MD; President Armed Forces Epidemiology Board and Friedman Professor of Pathology, Harvard University, Pathologist-in-Chief Peter Bent Brigham Hospital, Boston.

Robin D. Powell, MD; Clinical Director, Malaria Project, Assistant Professor of Medicine, The University of Chicago.

James V. McNamara, MD; Malaria Project.

Henri Frischer, MD, PhD; Assistant Professor of Medicine, The University of Chicago.

Leon O. Jacobson, MD; Dean of the Division of Biological Sciences & the School of Medicine, The University of Chicago.

Unknown.

Powell, MD, Shirley Hill, RN, Theodore N. Pullman, MD, Thomas Stockert, MD, Ann E. Lawrence, MD, Alvin R. Tarlov, MD, James E. Bowman, MD, Richard L. Landau, MD, and Henri Frischer, MD, PhD.

International Recognition of our Volunteers

Leonard J. Bruce-Chwatt, MD, the physician in charge of malaria research and control for the World Health Organization, an agency of the United Nations, wrote under **Letters** in *Science* 155: 1617-1618, 1967:

> "...I should like to stress how much medical science, and the human society as a whole, has benefited from investigations carried out on volunteers, deliberately infected with malaria, with the aim of assessing the value of various new drugs."

> "First of all it must be stated that no animal, with the exception of apes and monkeys, could be infected with human malaria parasites. Various experimental models on birds and rodents are useful only for preliminary screening of potentially valuable antimalarials."

> "...The decisive evaluation of drugs for the prevention and treatment of human malaria can be done only on man. For a number of years studies of antimalarial drugs were based upon the results of treatment of cases of malaria seen in hospitals. These observations were useful but the variability of the clinical response to natural malaria infections limited their scientific value and much difficulty has been experienced in the interpretation of data from different countries."

> "In 1942-43 when the acute shortage of quinine showed the vital need to develop new synthetic

drugs, a number of experimental studies were
carried out in Britain and the United States. The
most famous of these experiments were those by
Fairley in Australia on approximately 1000 army
volunteers deliberately infected with malaria. This
work was taken up in the United States by two
outstanding malaria research projects that started
in 1944 and still continue. One was set up at the
Federal Penitentiary in Atlanta (1), the other in
the Illinois State Penitentiary near Chicago (2).
The stated objective of both projects was to assess
the value of promising drugs for the prevention of
sporozoite-induced malaria and for the clinical and
radical cure of established infections. Those who
are acquainted not only with the rules governing
the acceptance of the service of volunteers in
these two research units, but also with the way
the medical and ethical principles are adhered to,
can bear testimony to the fact that the health, the
dignity, and freedom of choice of these subjects
were protected."

   "The World Organization expressed its appreciation of these studies in terms that are not often used in sober scientific reports (3)¶¶¶:
   "...At the present time, human malaria research
centres employing non-immune volunteers exist
only in the U.S.A. The amount and quality of
scientific data obtained in these centres on the
characteristics of drug-resistant strains of malaria
parasites and on their response to drugs is
invaluable, and...medical science owes an immense
debt of gratitude to the administrators of these

¶¶¶References: G.R. Coatney, W.C. Cooper, D.S. Ruhe, *Amer. J. Hyg.* **47**, 113
(1948); A.S. Alving, B. Craig, Jr., T.N. Pullman, C.M. Whorton, R. Jones, Jr., L.
Eichelberger; *J. Clin. Invest.* **27**, part 2, p. 2 (1948). *World Health Organ. Tech Rep.
Ser.* **296**, (1965).

institutions, to the research workers concerned, and above all to the courage and devotion of the volunteers."

"...It seems that straightforward, well-planned and perfectly executed investigations such as those at Atlanta and Stateville on fully informed, healthy human volunteers are ethically and professionally more justifiable than some trials done on hospital patients without their knowledge or consent."

L.J. Bruce-Chwatt, World Health Organization, Avenue Appia, 1211Geneva. Switzerland

Full Disclosure

Was there full disclosure of the studies we undertook with inmate volunteers in Stateville Penitentiary to find regimens to prevent and cure multi-drug resistant falciparum malaria? Yes.

My name appears as coauthor on 14 full-length papers published in peer-reviewed scientific journals from 1965-1967, in which we gave credit and thanks to the inmate volunteers who participated in the studies described therein: *Nature, Bulletin of the World Health Organization, American Journal of Tropical Medicine & Hygiene, Military Medicine, New England Journal of Medicine, International Journal of Leprosy, Annals of Tropical Medicine & Parasitology, and the Archives of Internal Medicine.*

Members of the Malaria Project gave oral presentations of our work at meetings of scientific societies in Rome, Chicago, New Orleans, Washington, D.C., and San Francisco, which were published as abstracts in *Journal of Laboratory Investigation, Journal of Clinical Investigation, Annals of Internal Medicine, Clinical Research*, and in the *Proceedings of the First International Congress of Parasitology.*

As fighting in Vietnam escalated, the American lay press reported on the morbidity from malaria in our combat troops and about
the success of our research findings at Stateville to prevent and cure
drug-resistant malaria.

Headlines told the story: "Army Seeks Antidote to Viet Malaria,"
Chicago Sun Times, 11APR1965; "Stamping Out Malaria," *Chicago
Tribune*, 20APR1965; "Malaria in Viet Nam," *Time*, 20AUG1965; "Bares
Quinine Shortage and Rise in Malaria," *Chicago Tribune*, 18NOV1965;
"High Viet Casualties Mean Work for Philippine Medics, *New York
Times*, 15NOV1965 and *Manila Times*, 25NOV1965; "Malaria Perils
Troops," *Indianapolis Star*, 25NOV1965; "Vietnam Type of Malaria is
Eased in Drug Tests," *New York Times*, 30NOV1965; "More Action,
More Malaria," *Time*, 10DEC1965; "GIs Fall Before New Viet Enemy-
Malaria, U. of C. Team Joins Army in Battle," *Chicago Daily News*,
11DEC1965; "Prisoners Help Test Drug for Malaria," *New York Times*,
16MAR1966; "Prison-Tested Drug Used in Viet Malaria War," *Chicago
Sun Times*, 16MAR1966; "New Malaria Drug Tested Effectively in S.
Vietnam," *Chicago Tribune*, 16MAR1966; "New Antimalarial Drug,"
University of Chicago Magazine, MAY1966; "Researchers Report
Breakthrough in Fight Against Malaria in Viet," *Iowa City Press-
Citizen*, 23JUN1966; "Volunteers Here Fight Malaria in Vital Battle of
Viet Nam War," *Joliet Herald-News*, Sunday, 20FEB1966; "1st Cavalry
Plagued by Malaria and Rats," *Chicago Tribune*, 11SEP1966; "Drug
May Cut Malaria Cases," *Des Moines Register*, 16OCT1966.

Recapitulation

We undertook clinical studies of malaria with inmate volunteers,
because our Commander-in-Chief, President Lyndon B. Johnson,

ordered U.S. Combat Troops into regions of endemic malaria in Vietnam, where multi-drug resistant *Plasmodium falciparum* malaria defied radical cure by Chloroquine and many other previously curative drugs.

Scientists in laboratories throughout the world had been unable to grow *P. falciparum* parasites, the malaria that infects human beings, in tissue culture or in non-immune animals. Drug studies in monkeys infected with *Plasmodium cynomolgi*, or in mice infected with *Plasmodium berghei,* failed to predict efficacy of the drugs in human beings. Moreover, observations of patients treated with malaria to abate the insanity of tertiary syphilis, and of patients naturally acquiring the disease, yielded equivocal results, unhelpful in developing regimens for the prevention and radical cure of multi-drug resistant malaria. Therefore, we carried out studies in healthy volunteer inmates in Illinois' maximum security prison, Stateville Penitentiary, to determine the efficacy and toxicity of drugs to prevent and cure mosquito-induced multi-drug resistant falciparum malaria, sensitive only to intravenously administered quinine sulfate, then in short supply outside of the Malaria Project.

For the safety of the volunteer, study participants were hospitalized and cared for by experienced physicians and nurses who relied on immediate laboratory support in the University of Chicago-Army Medical Research Project, a project with a 20-year record of safe operation. No inmate was coerced to volunteer, and all men participated after giving their informed consent verbally and in writing. Physician investigators and their staff adhered strictly to the rules of the Nuremberg Code for the safe conduct of experimental studies in human subjects. No permanent injuries or untoward events occurred during the studies.

At the time, there was full disclosure of the studies with oral presentations at national and international scientific meetings. Our regimens for the prevention and cure of multi-drug resistant falciparum malaria were adopted by the U.S. Army Medical Corps, and they were published in abstracts and full-length articles in the scientific literature. The contributions of our inmate volunteers were recognized, and they were reported with the results of our studies in local and nationally syndicated newspapers.

How could all of this come about? First, there was an urgent need to find prevention and cure of a disease affecting many persons, military and civilian. Second, the Malaria Project had the full support of the U.S. Army, The University of Chicago, and the State of Illinois. Third, Dr. Alving had directed the Project continuously for 20 years, recruiting well-trained medical officers whose terms of service overlapped, to provide more continuity. Fourth, a civilian nurse, with over a decade of service on the Project, supervised inmate nurses on the job 24/7. Fifth, technicians in the Project Laboratory were skilled and certified to provide immediate support for the clinical studies. Sixth, some members of the inmate staff had worked for many years on the Project , providing continuity by teaching new staff members. Seventh, the Project's location in the Prison Hospital meant that the prison physician, x-ray, and operating room facilities were close by on site. Finally, the success of the project was totally dependent upon healthy young men who had the initiative and courage to volunteer for the studies undertaken.

GOOD HART

Mixed aromas from a wood fire in the stone fireplace, and from scrambled eggs and bacon on the kitchen range, awakened Karen and me on a cool summer morning. Mother was cooking breakfast.

Bobby, two years old in a couple of months, snoozed in a crib at the foot of our bed. We were guests of my parents in a cottage on the eastern shore of beautiful Lake Michigan. They had rented this cottage in Good Hart, Michigan, for the month of August 1964.

Robin had urged me to take a week's leave after having taken call 24/7 on the Project during the first three weeks in July until my new partner, Ben Eppes, completed his training at Fort Sam Houston and reported for duty at the end of the month. As the new co-director, Robin frequently visited the Project in July, but he proposed to be on site every day while I was gone, so he could work closely with Ben, bringing him "up to speed" as my full partner by the time I returned.

Located in the woods just south of Mackinaw City and the Straits of Mackinac, in the northern tip of mainland Michigan, Good Hart boasted a general store/post office, gasoline pumps, and an antique shop. We had almost missed the turn off state road #119, which led down a gravel road to the lake, and then on a one-lane road through the woods to the cottage. My parents greeted us warmly on our arrival. My mother took Bobby's hand, showing him the cottage, and then took him out its front door to view, through stately conifers, sandy beaches and sparkling Lake Michigan, where in the days to come he would wade, swim, and explore the beach for shells and Petoskey Stones with his grandmother.

Nellie and Cliff Powers ran the store/post office at Good Hart. My father and I arrived at the store/post office about 11:00 a.m., when shortly thereafter, an old 2-door sedan with three persons in it, parked in front of the store. A young Native American climbed out of the driver's seat, opened the car's trunk, extracted an official-looking canvass mail bag, lugged it into the store, and dumped it in the middle of the floor for Cliff to distribute its contents to the pigeon holes behind the counter. When my father asked the postman about the elderly man and woman, staring straight ahead, sitting motionless in the back seat of his car, he replied, "Oh, they are my parents. If I don't take them on the route with me, they will be drunk before noon."

My father and I anxiously retrieved from the mail delivery at the store, the package containing galley proofs of chapters of *Bedside Diagnostic Examination* (BDE 1/e), sent by **Joan C. Zulch**, Editor-in-Chief, Medical Books Department, Macmillan Publishing Company, New York. Earlier that morning, we had reviewed final drafts and galleys of early chapters of the book my father had written with my assistance. It instructed medical students and practicing physicians on how to take a history, perform a physical examination, select appropriate laboratory tests, and devise a differential diagnosis in order to reach a definitive diagnosis of a patient's illness. At the time, we had no idea that by the publication of its third edition, BDE 3/e, in 1976, it would have been adopted by all medical schools in the United States, half the Canadian medical schools, schools of Osteopathy, schools of nursing, and Physician Assistant programs. Whereas eight competing textbooks on physical diagnosis soon went out of print, *DeGowin's Diagnostic Examination* (10/e) (I had changed the name), has remained in print for over a half-century.

1964—CIVIL WAR CENTENNIAL

One hundred years after a bloody Civil War that ended black slavery in the South, in which my Great-Grandfather, **Henry DeGowin,** fought in Company D, 142nd New York Volunteer Infantry to free the slaves, black citizens of the United States still suffered the humiliation of segregation and discrimination.

By 1865, some 800,000 American young men had lost their lives, the result of a war started by Southern Democrats who opposed the election of the first Republican President of the United States,

Abraham Lincoln. Within six months of their surrender, unrepentant rebels rallied in Pulaski, Tennessee, on the day before Christmas, to follow slave-master **Nathan Bedford Forest**, founding leader of the Ku Klux Klan, to terrorize black citizens who would vote for Republican candidates for office.

Federal troops sent to the South to secure voting rights for all citizens, guaranteed by Amendment XIII of the U.S. Constitution, were withdrawn in 1877 at the close of Reconstruction, permitting Southern Democrats to further intimidate and suppress black Americans. President **Woodrow Wilson**, a Virginia Democrat, upheld laws segregating blacks in the public places of our nation's Capital during his administration, 1913-1921.

In 1953, during his first year in office, Republican President **Dwight David Eisenhower** desegregated Washington, D.C. by executive order. On 17 May 1954, the U.S. Supreme Court ruled unanimously in *Brown vs. Board of Education of Topeka* that racial segregation in public schools was unconstitutional. Defying the ruling on 4 September 1957, Governor **Orval Faubus** ordered the Arkansas National Guardsmen to bar nine black students from entering the all-white Little Rock High School. Unable to convince the grand-standing Democrat Governor of Arkansas to enforce integration, on 24 September 1957 President Eisenhower dispatched 1,000 soldiers of the famous 101st Airborne Division to ensure that the *Little Rock Nine* were admitted to Little Rock High School.

On 1 December 1955, **Rosa Parks**, a black woman, refused to relinquish her seat in the back of a municipal bus to a white man in Montgomery, Alabama. A Federal Court declared the bus segregation ordinance unconstitutional following a boycott of the bus system by blacks in Montgomery, organized and led by Reverend Martin Luther King, Jr.

Dr. Martin Luther King, Jr. thrilled a crowd of 250,000 people during his *March on Washington,* and he entranced a vast television audience as he declared, "I have a dream.." in his famous speech, delivered from the steps of the Lincoln Memorial on 24 August 1963. In his speech he envisioned a "color-blind" society where each person was judged on their character and merit.

He received the Nobel Peace Prize on 10 December 1964, and he was assassinated in Memphis, Tennessee, on 4 April 1968.

Civil Rights

BLACK MUSLIMS

When Karen and I married, our first apartment was at #708, 727 East 60th Street, in an integrated building on Chicago's South Side. Of its 320 apartments, only 10 were occupied by white residents. Consequently, we received radical literature directed at our black neighbors. My first encounter with a Black Muslim occurred when a representative of Elijah Muhammad knocked on my door selling a newspaper, *Muhammad Speaks*. After he recovered from the shock of being greeted by a resident with a very pale face, he sold me the paper. It was filled with propaganda about the candidates for the election that fall of 1962.

Elijah Muhammad (1897-1975), leader of the Black Muslims from 1934 to 1975, established the University of Islam for black children several blocks north of The University of Chicago Campus. Elijah preached political, social, and economic independence for Black Americans. As black pride emerged during the 1950's and 60's, many blacks embraced Islam, changed their Anglo names to Arabic and joined the Muslims. Most notable, a boxer named for a Kentucky abolitionist, **Cassius M. Clay**, won the World Boxing Association (WBA) Heavyweight Championship by defeating Sonny Liston in 1964. He defended his title until he received his draft notice. Then

Clay changed his name to **Muhammad Ali** and refused military induction on "religious grounds," and the WBA vacated his title in 1967. Ironically, his namesake, Cassius Marcellus Clay, served as Major General of Union Volunteers in the Civil War, ending black slavery in the United States.

"Reveal Stateville Revolt by Four Black Muslims," *Chicago Tribune*, 4 July 1964. On 22 June 1964, the U.S. Supreme Court ruled that lower courts erred in dismissing a suit by Thomas Cooper 32, a Black Muslim murderer confined to the Segregation Unit in Stateville, in which he claimed prison authorities had violated his rights by refusing to allow him to practice his religion. The high tribunal ordered the Federal District Court to investigate Cooper's claim.

Later in June, four other Black Muslim prisoners incarcerated for murder, rape, and robbery—serving time in Segregation, because they could not live peaceably with other inmates—presented lengthy written demands to Warden Frank J. Pate, insisting that they be permitted to leave their cells 6-7 times daily to pray in the Prison Chapel, that they be assigned a special cook to prepare special food for them, and that they be allowed to distribute (inflammatory) Black Muslim literature among fellow prisoners.

After their demands were rejected on 2 July 1964, they threw urine and feces on their guards. One excited prisoner broke out the ½-inch thick glass in his cell's overhead light fixture and yelled, "Come on in and get me!" He tried to slash Assistant Warden Revis and other officers with a razor-sharp shard of broken glass from the light fixture as they pushed him to the back of his cell behind a large Plexiglas shield. As he thrashed around the edge of the shield, he slipped on his own urine, fell, and cut his scalp on the toilet fixture. The scalp laceration bled profusely for a minute or two.

Call the Malaria Doc

In the absence of the prison physician, Dr. Julius Venckus, who was in Joliet at the time, Assistant Warden Revis called the Malaria Doc, me, to the Isolation Office at 3:15 pm 2 July 1964 to provide medical care for the now subdued rebels. Warden Pate, having joined us, told each man standing in front of us, "Captain DeGowin is a medical doctor here to help you. Tell him if you are not feeling well." All but one said they, "felt well."

Morris, for whom I use a fictional name, said that he was a little weak in his legs. Yet, he stood and walked without difficulty. Except for a scalp laceration on his right occipital area, my examination revealed no neurological deficits or other abnormalities. His scalp wound was slightly tender, but there was no sign of skull fracture. Morris had not lost consciousness when he fell in his cell hitting his head on the toilet, but Warden Pate, cognizant of the litigation in which these inmates were engaged, asked, "Doc, wouldn't you like to have skull x-rays on this man?" "Yes!" I replied without hesitation.

After obtaining the skull x-rays, which were normal, Morris sat calmly on the x-ray machine table. I cleaned his wound with soap and water and closed the small (1.0 cm) superficial laceration with two silk sutures. All the while, Morris had been talking to the wardens, when in a genuinely sympathetic tone, Warden Revis asked, "What got into you, Morris?" Morris answered, "I don't know, Warden. I jus' got stoomoolated."

President Barack Hussein Obama

Martin Luther King, Jr., did not survive to celebrate the election on 4 November 2008 of **Barack Hussein Obama**, the first black president of the United States. Reminding us of Obama's roots in Chicago politics, Illinois Governor **Rod Blagojevich**, impeached for corruption and for attempting to sell Obama's vacated seat in the U.S. Senate, was discharged from office on 29 January 2009 by a vote of 59-0 in the Illinois Senate. Potential appointees to the seat in the Senate included Jesse Jackson, Jr. and **Valerie B. Jarrett**. Valerie Jarrett, daughter of my good friend Jim Bowman, withdrew her name from consideration. She served as senior adviser to the president for all eight years of the Obama Administration, the longest such service in history.

University of Chicago Magazine, Jan-Feb 2009, arrived in my mail 30 January 2009 with a story about Obama's staff with University of Chicago connections:

> "First up was Obama campaign adviser and transition-team co-chair Valerie B. Jarrett, joining the White House Staff as senior adviser, assistant to the president for intergovernmental relations and public liaison. Jarrett, who chairs the Medical Center's trustees and is vice chair of the University Board of Trustees, met Obama in 1991, when she was Chicago Mayor Richard M. Daley's deputy chief of staff. She has even stronger ties to the University. Her father, **James Bowman**, is professor emeritus in pathology and medicine, and her mother, **Barbara Taylor Bowman**, AM'52, who taught at the Lab Schools, where Jarrett was a student is an early-childhood-education expert who cofounded the Erickson Institute."

Walter Reed Army Institute of Research (WRAIR)

Antimalarial Vaccine

Scientists at Walter Reed Army Institute of Research (WRAIR) proposed to make a vaccine to prevent multi-drug resistant falciparum malaria from infecting our troops in Vietnam by injecting the human malaria into chimpanzees, which had undergone splenectomy to lower their immune system, making them better hosts for malaria parasites that exclusively infected human beings.

Shortly after the New Year, I was riding in a taxi in downtown Chicago, bound for the airport. The elderly cabbie, noting my uniform said, "I was working here in December, and I hadn't seen so many troops going through town since World War II!" Sure enough, President Johnson had done exactly what he had accused his campaign opponent, Senator Barry Goldwater of planning, and what Johnson had said he would never do—escalate the war in Vietnam.

Later, I learned why I was the chosen courier. But here I was in January 1965 on a United Airlines Flight from O'Hare International Airport to Washington National Airport (now Reagan National Airport). Between my knees, I gingerly carried an iced thermos bottle containing mosquito salivary glands, infected with sporozoites from the multi-drug resistant Malayan (Camp) strain of *P. falciparum*, that Robin, Jerry, and I had painstakingly dissected from female *Anopheles stephensi* in the Insectary at Stateville earlier that day.

Robin and other malariologists thought that inducing immunity to sporozoites, the first stage of the malaria infection, would prove more effective than trying to suppress later stages of an established infection. They were 40 years ahead of their time. Our attempt to develop a vaccine against malarial sporozoites failed, but later studies provided a ray of hope: "Malaria vaccine shows promise in Africa tests."[****]

[****] The Gazette, p. 5, 9DEC2008; Bejon, P. et al: Efficacy of RTS, S/AS01E Vaccine against Malaria in Children 5 to17 Months of Age, N. Engl. J. Med. 359:2521-2532, 11DEC2008; Collins, W.E. & Barnwell, J.W.: A Hopeful Beginning for Malaria Vaccines, N. Engl. J. Med. 359, 2599-2600, 11DEC2008.

COLONEL WILLIAM CROSBY, MC

After depositing the thermos bottle in the hands of waiting scientists at WRAIR, I was introduced to the renowned hematologist **Colonel William Crosby, MC**, and to his genial staff of physician-scientist medical officers. A kind man and thoughtful host, whose scientific work I had followed and admired in the medical literature, Dr. Crosby showed me around his impressive and well-equipped laboratory. At the end of our tour, he turned and asked me if I would like to join his research group at the conclusion of my duty at Stateville in July 1965. Needless to say, I was taken aback by this flattering job offer. As we walked down the corridor to meet his boss, Colonel William Tigertt, I mumbled something about continuity of duty station if I stayed in the Army.

COLONEL WILLIAM D. TIGERTT, MC, COMMANDANT, WALTER REED ARMY INSTITUTE OF RESEARCH

He was slender, fit, and unsmiling, sitting in uniform behind a large desk, resting upon which, was a rectangular plaque imprinted with: **"Colonel William D. Tigertt, MC."** Frontal balding left a dark patch of hair in the center above his forehead. Tinged with gray, it matched the configuration and coloring of his mustache. His unblinking gaze fixed on me as he peered over the top of reading glasses and asked Colonel Crosby, coming right to the point, "Well, Bill, does DeGowin want to join us here in July?" Dr. Crosby replied, "He says that he is impressed with our staff and the facilities, but he is concerned that he might have to interrupt a research project if, as an Army Officer, he was transferred to another assignment."

There followed a tense and lengthy silence as Colonel Tigertt stared at the ceiling. (Some of his subordinates dropped the last two t's in his name when they spoke of him out of earshot.) Then he drilled Colonel Crosby with a penetrating expression and asked, "How long have you been here, Bill?" In deference, Dr. Crosby replied, "Fourteen years, Sir." Within a year or so of that response, Bill Crosby had resigned his commission and taken the job as Director of Hematology at Tufts University Medical Center in Boston.

THE MEETING OF 24 MAY 1965

The next time I saw Colonel Tigertt was 41 days before my separation from the U.S. Army. I am looking at a photograph taken on 24 May 1965 in the Malaria Project Conference Room. Robin Powell had invited ten of us to review our data on the prevention and cure of multi-drug resistant falciparum malaria. Action, taken as a result of our discussion of the data, depended upon the decision of one participant sitting at our conference table, **Colonel William D. Tigertt**.

Seated at the table on the left of Colonel Tigertt is **Robin D. Powell, MD**, Assistant Professor of Medicine, University of Chicago (UC), and Co-Director, Army Medical Research Project (AMRP), Stateville Penitentiary. On Dr. Tigertt's right sits an alumnus of the Malaria Project, and former teacher of Robin and me, **John D. Arnold, MD**, Chairman of Internal Medicine, University of Missouri-Kansas City, and Director of The Harry Truman Laboratories. John had developed a malaria project with inmate volunteers in the Kansas City Jackson County Jail.

Standing behind the table from left to right: **Leon H. Schmidt, PhD**, Director, National Primate Center, University of California-Davis, and Chairman, Commission on Malaria, Armed Forces Epidemiological Board; **Peter G. Contacos, MD**, Head of Cytology Laboratory, Parasite Chemotherapy, NIH, formerly clinical head of the NIH Malaria Unit, Federal Penitentiary, Atlanta, Georgia; **G. Robert Coatney, PhD**, Chief, Laboratory of Parasite Chemotherapy,

NIH, Bethesda, Maryland; and **Paul E. Carson, MD**, Assistant Professor, UC, and Co-Director AMRP, Stateville Penitientiary, discoverer of glucose-6-phosphate dehydrogenase in primaquine-sensitive red blood cells.

Standing next to Paul are the only two men in uniform: **Captain R. Bennett Eppes, MC** (my partner), Research Assistant, UC; **Captain Richard L. DeGowin, MC**, Research Associate, UC; and to my left is **Donald McMullen, PhD**, Scientist Advisor, WRAIR, Washington, D.C.

The Decision

It became clear from the remarks from various members of the group that President Johnson's deployment in Vietnam of more U.S. Combat Troops, resulted in more soldiers becoming infected with falciparum malaria, resistant to Chloroquine and other standard antimalarial drugs.

They agreed there was a desperate need to prevent and cure multidrug resistant falciparum malaria. After we presented our data on the prevention in non-immune volunteers of mosquito-induced drug resistant malaria with Diaminodiphenyl Sulfone (DDS), and reviewed our results in curing the infections with Pyrimethamine-Sulfadiazine (a similar combination of drugs, based on our work, was later produced commercially as *Fansidar*, used to cure multi-drug resistant falciparum malaria in civilians throughout the tropics), there followed a tense silence. Then all members of the group looked at Colonel Tigertt, who smiled and said, "**Let's go with it!**" That meant within a few weeks, the U.S. Army Medical Corps would introduce into field trials in Vietnam, the drug regimens we had developed on the Malaria Project at Stateville. Wow! Mission Accomplished!

A year and a half later, I received a letter from the former Surgeon General, my boss:

Fitzsimmons General Hospital
Denver, Colorado 80240
Office of the Commanding General

6 January 1967

Richard L. DeGowin, MD
Assistant Professor of Medicine
Argonne Cancer Research Hospital
950 East 59th Street
Chicago, Illinois 60637

Dear Doctor DeGowin:
Many thanks for the reprints in addition to the WHO/Mal series reports of some of your studies. Thanks to your efforts the DDS is apparently proving helpful in reducing the morbidity in malaria.

It appears that more and more cases of vivax are turning up; at least at the 85th Evacuation Hospital at Qui Nhon. The explanation is not yet clear.

Sincerely,

Robert E. Blount
Major General MC
Commanding

Framed, the letter hung on my office wall for many years.

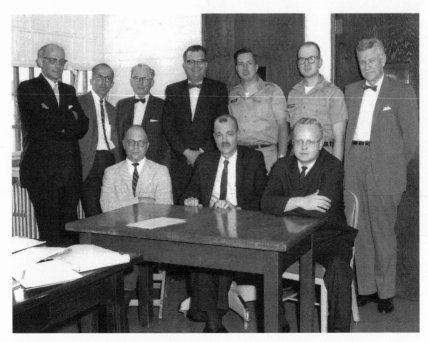

The Decision, Stateville, 24May1965, [Seated (l.-r.)]:

John D. Arnold, MD; Chairman, Internal Medicine, The University of Missouri-Kansas City.

Colonel William D. Tigertt, MC; Commandant, Walter Reed Army Institute of Research.

Robin D. Powell, MD; Clinical Director, Malaria Project, Stateville; Assistant Professor of Medicine, The University of Chicago.

[Standing (l.-r.)]:

Leon H. Schmidt, PhD; Chairman, Malaria Commission, Armed Forces Epidemiological Board; Director, National Primate Center, The University of California-Davis.

Peter G. Contacos, MD; Head of Cytology Laboratory, Parasite Chemotherapy, NIH; Former Clinical Head of NIH Malaria Unit, Federal Penitentiary, Atlanta, Georgia.

G. Robert Coatney, PhD; Chief, Laboratory of Parasite Chemotherapy, NIH, Bethesda, Maryland.

Paul E. Carson, MD; Scientific Director, Malaria Project, Stateville. Assistant Professor of Medicine, The University of Chicago; Discovered glucose-6-dehydrogenase deficiency in primaquine-sensitive red blood cells.

Captain R. Bennett Eppes, MC; Stateville, Research Assistant, The University of Chicago.

Captain Richard L. DeGowin, MC; Stateville, Research Associate, The University of Chicago.

Donald McMullen, PhD; Scientist Advisor, Walter Reed Army Institute of Research

Part IV. The Job
(1965)

Interviews

Karen agreed with me. At age 31, after 8 years of marital bliss, the blessings of a 2-½ year old healthy son, 11 years of advanced education after high school, and 2 years' active duty in the Army, it was time to get a real job. I had declined an offer to retain my Captain's Commission and accept a good position with Colonel William Crosby's research group at Walter Reed Army Institute of Research. But in complaining to my mentor and friend, **Dr. Clifford W. Gurney**, about the "publish or perish" pressures and the politics associated with a tenure-track post in academic medicine, I said I was inclined to apply for a job in a Veterans Hospital, where I could see patients and do research, instead of returning to The University of Chicago in Cliff's Division of Hematology. Cliff said, "You don't want to do that!"

Shortly thereafter, I received letters from hematologists at The University of Louisville, at The University of Michigan, and at The University of Illinois inviting me to interview for a position in their sections of hematology. Without telling me about it, Cliff had bragged about me to his acquaintances from these other schools of medicine, resulting in three opportunities to interview for a job. What a nice guy!

Giovanni Raccuglia, MD, met me at the airport in Louisville, Kentucky. I had never been to Kentucky before. Dr. Raccuglia, Director of Hematology, was a slender dark-haired man in his early 40's. He proudly showed me around the hospital, a large old city-run institution wherein clinical teaching for The University of Louisville Medical School took place. I remembered The University of Cincinnati was the only other medical school that used exclusively a municipal hospital for clinical teaching, a red flag right there. I knew how the Democrat machine ran Cook County Hospital in Chicago with patronage jobs to pay off the party faithful, whose mission sometimes failed to coincide with that of the medical faculty of the schools that used County Hospital for clinical teaching of medical students and house staff.

In the office of the Department of Internal Medicine, Dr. Raccuglia introduced me to its chairman, **Dr. Beverly Robetson**, silver mane, not a hair out of place, chiseled facial features, smoking a black pipe clenched in a strong jaw, black suit, and a soft Southern accent. He was cordial, but cool. On our way to his home for a reception in late afternoon, Dr. Raccuglia, a blood clotting specialist, recalled for me his fellowship in hematology and junior faculty position at The University of Michigan. That is where he met Cliff Gurney, who was in residency and fellowship training at Michigan then. So that was Cliff's connection. Dr. Raccuglia was the only member of his Section of Hematology at Louisville, which, like many other medical schools in the 1960's, was expanding its faculty to meet the need for more doctors. He and Dr. Robertson offered me a position with the rank of Instructor. I declined, looking for a job as assistant professor where I could have research time, sharing call with several colleagues.

Many fond memories of good times flooded my consciousness in my return to Ann Arbor. I remembered accompanying, as a young child, my mother and father, alumni of The University of Michigan, when they visited Aunt Frances and Uncle Rob in their home at 519 Lawrence Street. There, I enjoyed reunions with cousins, aunts and uncles, who had graduated from Michigan. I recalled the good friends, roommates in South Quadrangle, and with whom I had walked to my premedical classes at The University of Michigan from the fall of 1952 until the spring of 1955. Of the three medical schools where I was accepted, Michigan was my second choice. But I was fortunate to be accepted at The University of Chicago where I spent ten years in one or another capacity. It would have proved difficult for both my father and me if I attended The University of Iowa, where Dad taught in the College of Medicine.

The Simpson Memorial Institute, a four story neoclassic structure across Observatory Drive from The University of Michigan Hospitals, was built in the 1920's with a gift from its namesake to discover a cure for pernicious anemia. Shortly before construction was finished, however, liver extract, then Vitamin B12, proved effective therapies to impart a healthy normal life span for patients faced with death from a lethal nutritional deficiency. Now, this whole building served as home to the Division of Hematology, including their clinics, beds, laboratories and offices. Recently renovated, it provided unique facilities for hematology faculty members.

My host, **Christopher Zarafanetis, MD**, Director of Hematology, trim, of medium height, closely cropped gray hair, rimless glasses, courteous, and kind, introduced me to the other members of his division. We made rounds on their patients in University Hospitals, and then we attended the Hematology Fellows' Journal Club meeting. One of the fellows, a foreign medical graduate, proceeded to critically review a journal article he had selected without making the connection with the name of the lead author: DeGowin, R.L. & Gurney, C.W.: Hemopoiesis in Polycythemia Vera After Phlebotomy and Iron Therapy,. *Arch. Intern. Med.* 114:424-433, 1964. He proceeded to tear to shreds one of my favorite papers, alleging that the authors' speculation, which Cliff and I had clearly labeled as such, was totally unjustified by the results of the clinical studies we had described in the article. Amazingly, the fellow did not realize the lead author, yours truly, was sitting across the conference table from him, but Chris Zarafanetis did, was embarrassed for me, and apologized for the fellow's insensitive remarks. By the way, our observations were accurate and our speculation proved true in studies by other investigators.

I cannot recall if my discussion with Dr. Zarafanetis regarding the position of Assistant Professor at Michigan, a much better opportunity than that offered at Louisville, continued beyond the first interview, but I looked to a future interview at The University of Illinois.

THE UNIVERSITY OF ILLINOIS

I had met my host **Dr. Paul Heller**, at hematology meetings, and I knew of his excellent research on sickle cell anemia, undertaken with hematology fellows in his productive laboratory in the Westside Veterans Administration Hospital. Affiliated with The University of Illinois Medical School, the Westside VA was less than a block from the Illinois Research & Education Hospital (Illinois R&E) and a block from the massive Cook County Hospital, just west of downtown Chicago, off the Eisenhower Expressway. Illinois R&E was the main teaching hospital for The University of Illinois.

As I recall Paul Heller, he was a man of medium height and build with a shock of black hair and a German accent. Much later I learned that his experience as a young man in the 1930's and 40's involved the medical care of Jewish prisoners in a Nazi Concentration Camp, where he was imprisoned. He was a Holocaust survivor. I remember him as a brilliant, warm, and kind man. Dr. Heller, whom years later I called "Paul," showed me his laboratory, the clinics and the laboratories in the Illinois R&E Hospital, where he bought me lunch in the cafeteria. A couple of other hematologists on the faculty joined us for introductions and conversation. In early afternoon, after more discussion, Dr. Heller ushered me into the office of the Chairman of Internal Medicine, **Harry F. Dowling, MD**.

Seated behind a large wooden desk in his big office, Dr. Dowling stood, smiled, and shook my hand firmly. He was of average height and weight, balding, wearing spectacles, reminding me a little of Chris Zarafanetis. In addition to Dr. Dowling's administrative responsibilities, he practiced as an infectious disease specialist, and remarked about my work on malaria. As we talked, I came to realize he was offering me a tenure-track appointment as Assistant Professor of Medicine and to be the Director of Hematology at Illinois R&E Hospital. I tried to conceal my surprise.

In response to his question, "What will you need to come here?" I replied, "Well, I will need a laboratory, with basic equipment, an office, etc." Then he leaned forward and asked, "Yes, of course, but what annual salary would you need?" Boy! I wasn't ready for that one. I paused to think for a moment. I thought I should ask for more money than I was making in the Army as a Captain in the Medical Corps at $10,000 a year, so I said, "$12,000 per year." There followed palpable silence. Then Dr. Dowling got up from his desk, smiled, shook my hand again, and said, "I will call you within the week."

After leaving Dr. Dowling's office, I stopped to see a friend, a rheumatologist on the Illinois faculty, who warned me the State of Illinois had been frugal to penurious in funding its medical school in Chicago. He told me that faculty salaries fell below those at The University of Chicago and other medical schools in the Midwest.

After relating my interview with Harry Dowling at Illinois R&E to Cliff Gurney in his office at the Argonne Cancer Research Hospital (ACRH) at The University of Chicago, where Cliff was Director of Hematology, Cliff said, but not in these words that I inferred, "Dummy! You never tell them what salary you want. Make them make an offer. It might be higher than your figure."

The University of Chicago

I had taken for granted the facilities the Section of Hematology faculty members in the Department of Internal Medicine enjoyed with their appointments on the staff of the **Argonne Cancer Research Hospital (ACRH).** Attached by corridors to The University of Chicago Hospitals and Clinics, the six floors of the ACRH contained two inpatient units for hematology and oncology patients, research and clinical laboratories, a conference room, administrative and editorial offices, animal care facilities, radiation facilities, an isotope manufacturing pharmacy, a machine shop for building laboratory instruments, and a cyclotron in the basement.

Dr. Leon O. "Jake" Jacobson served as Director of ACRH, as well as Chairman of the Department of Internal Medicine, Cliff Gurney's boss. He operated ACRH with a generous annual grant from the U.S. Atomic Energy Commission in a program to study the peaceful use of atoms and radiation in the treatment of patients with cancer and other diseases. Including Jake, who continued to see his hematology patients in addition to his administrative duties, there were six physicians in Cliff Gurney's Section of Hematology, which occupied research laboratories and offices on the entire second floor of the ACRH. The grant paid for their salaries, salaries for their research assistants, and purchased laboratory instruments, equipment, and research supplies. If they failed to produce, they lost their appointment and had to move out.

Of course, I knew, admired, and liked all the members of the Section of Hematology, having worked in Cliff's research lab on the second floor before I went in the Army. Four became Chairmen of Departments of Internal Medicine: Dr. Jacobson (who later became Dean of The University of Chicago School of Medicine), Al Tarlov, Dick Blaisdell, and Cliff Gurney.

Good to his word, Dr. Dowling called me back to his office at Illinois R&E later in the week. He smiled and said, "Dr. DeGowin, we would very much like to have you join us." I had a job! "But," he went on, "we cannot afford to pay you an annual salary of $12,000." I didn't have a job! Later I learned that one of Paul Heller's former hematology fellows took the job for $9,000 per year. Of course, my classmates who entered the private practice of medicine cleared four to five times the income I had requested for a job in academic medicine.

ACRH

In one day, I went from being unemployed to have the best job I could have imagined. Cliff Gurney had gone to Jake and said, "Dr. Jacobson, as I build this Section of Hematology, I will need three new Assistant Professors: Sandy Krantz (my classmate), Wally Fried, and Dick DeGowin. Wally will be here for six months before he joins the faculty at Rush Medical School, but I will need appointments and laboratories in the ACRH for Sandy and Dick with an annual salary of $12,000 for each. DeGowin has already had four interviews for jobs elsewhere."

Jake said, "O.K."

Cliff said, "Dick, you start the first of July as Assistant Professor of Medicine in Hematology with an appointment as Project Supervisor in ACRH and a salary $12,000 per year. Do you want the job?" Without hesitation, I said, "Yes, I do, and thank you!"

Epilogue: A Goal of Self-Control

Of the 18 inmates who served as our staff on the Malaria Project at Stateville, none had attended college, and some had failed to graduate from high school. Yet, they performed as clerks, nurses, and skilled laboratory technicians in a manner equal or better than their counterparts with whom I had worked outside prison. These men, murderers, rapists, thieves, certified by the State of Illinois, had lacked the self-control to obey the law, but performed exceptionally well when the state imposed control.

In a remarkable study, a law-abiding normal citizen and a murderer were confronted with a scenario requiring self-control of the subject. A P.E.T. scan (Positron Emission Tomography) of each man showed markedly increased metabolic activity in the frontal cortex of the brain (the seat of self-control) in the normal citizen, but none in the brain of the murderer. We were not told if the citizen learned self-control over the 18 years he might have spent in a family with a loving mother and father, who taught him right from wrong, enhancing the circuitry in his frontal cortex, and if the murderer lacked such an upbringing.

Having lived in Chicago's South Side, where the boys of fatherless families shoot each other every day, I recall an admonition by President Barack Obama, who declared when he was running for office, that men should take responsibility and act like fathers instead of boys, regarding the children born and raised out of wedlock. Is it unreasonable to assume that it is difficult, if not impossible, for a mother to work at a job to provide for her children while she needs to instill a sense of self-control in her boys without her husband's help as a disciplinarian and role-model of self-control?

Kings in ancient times, through the 19th century, imposed control of their subjects to live in peace with each other. During the 20th and 21st centuries, dictators of fascist regimes, arising from socialism, like the National Socialist Workers' Party (Hitler's Nazis), and like the Union of Soviet Socialist Republics (Stalin's USSR), disciplined their people, or like Stalin did, killed them if they didn't behave.

By contrast, in an era of kings where the state controlled its people, our founding fathers brought forth a nation in which the American citizens controlled the government. John Adams warned that without religion to instill self-discipline; i.e., self-control in the citizen living free in a Democratic Republic, the United States would soon perish. If a society is to be free of chaos, the person living in a free country must respect the rights of his fellow citizens.

The thousands of refugees seeking asylum in the United States, appearing at our southern border, bear testimony that a state that fails to enforce the rule of law, as in some countries in Central and South America, does not provide the benefits of a peaceful community for its honest citizens.

In 1963, the Malaria Docs and their wives—Julie and Robin, Karen and I—were invited to join administrative staff, wardens, guards, clerks and their families at Stateville's annual Christmas party in a rented hall in Joliet. We enjoyed Christmas music, good food, and dancing, in a relaxed setting, free from the tension we experienced working behind bars. I am not sure what I expected, but I was pleased to hear the after dinner remarks of Warden Frank Pate, who encouraged those present to help the prison inmates "do time," and improve their lives by advancing their education in school, learning skills in the vocational school, and/or acquiring a work ethic in the prison industries. In a sense, he was urging us to help these men acquire the self-control they needed to function successfully in society once released from prison.

You might ask how the total control of an inmate's behavior by the prison system could enhance his self-control, permitting him to live with other persons without killing, assaulting, or stealing from them. Incentives to acquire self-discipline were offered the inmate in a series of steps, each step granting him greater freedom from supervision and control by others. Violent inmates were placed in Isolation, a cell with a blanket, food, and sensory deprivation, for no more than a maximum of eleven days. The next steps were Segregation, like a county jail cell, then to the Cell Blocks and the Yard with a cellmate, the greater freedom all dependent upon the inmate's acquiring the self-control permitting him to live peacefully among others. Greater freedom and trust came with assignment for work in the Administration Building, its offices, the hospital, "up front," and finally, outside the walls on the Honor Farm.

In addition to providing incentives for the inmate to acquire self-control, the staff at Stateville offered programs to help an inmate rejoin society as a contributing member when released from prison. If he was illiterate, he could learn to read and lacking a high school diploma, he could attend prison school to receive his G.E.D. (General Equivalency Diploma), and even credits for the first three years of college. He could learn a skill in the vocational school, necessary to obtain a meaningful job, and acquire a work ethic in the prison industries. Even with all of these opportunities to improve his situation, over half of the inmates discharged from prison were later incarcerated again. Obviously, more help for inmates after their release from prison was needed to reduce a 50% rate of recidivism.

For those convicts needing more supervision after discharge, consider how the Civilian Conservation Corps (CCC), served inmates discharged from prison during the Great Depression. They worked outside in a unit run with the discipline of a military company, improving our country's infrastructure. Now they could live in barracks or townhouses, as in a company town, monitored with electronic bracelets or implanted chips to locate their movements, providing some exterior control until an individual proved he could function well without it.

A Parole Board with expanded duties and consultants could determine whether a convict had assumed enough self-control to advance to greater freedom from living with supervision and discipline imposed by the state. The consultants, active or retired, serving on the Parole Board might include a psychiatrist, a pastor, a social worker, a high school principal, and a law enforcement officer. Tests of convicts, based upon research derived from P.E.T. scanning of the brain's frontal cortex, might help members of the Board decide how much freedom to recommend for a former inmate. I suppose all of this depends upon whether society favors rehabilitation over revenge and punishment.

Appendix One

It was only after serving on active duty as Captain in the U.S. Army Medical Corps that I began to appreciate the outstanding contributions of military medicine to civilian health care.

Of course, I was aware of the research on the preservation, transportation, and transfusion of whole blood for the treatment of hemorrhagic shock undertaken shortly before (1938-1941), and during World War II (1941-1945), by my father, Elmer L. DeGowin (1901-1980). Serving on the National Research Council, he had successfully advocated for the use of whole blood, instead of plasma, to treat hemorrhagic shock arising from battlefield wounds. Results of his work facilitated the development of blood banks that supported surgical and obstetrical procedures in civilian medical practice in the United States and abroad.

Like Ambroise Pare (1510-1590), the "Father of Surgery," many surgeons developed skills, later used in civilian practice, by operating on battlefield casualties. Napoleon's Surgeon-in-Chief of the *Grand Armee*, Baron Dominque Jean Larrey (1766-1842), introduced in 1792, *ambulances volantes* (flying ambulances), sprung two-wheeled enclosed carts pulled by two fleet horses, to rapidly carry wounded men from the front lines of the battlefield to hospitals in the rear for definitive care. Motorized ambulances in World War I (1916-1918) and World War II (1941-1945) were supplanted by helicopter evacuation of American wounded men in the Korean War (1950-1953), and in the Vietnam War (1961-1973). These latter experiences provided the protocols and pilots for the transport of civilian patients by helicopter, commonly seen at most large tertiary medical care centers in the 21st century.

TRANSLATIONAL RESEARCH

Dr. William Beaumont (1785-1853), a U.S. Army Surgeon, carried out the first definitive studies of gastric physiology on his patient, Alexis St. Martin. St. Martin, a French-Canadian voyageur, survived a shotgun blast to his abdomen in 1822 at the American Fur Company Office in Fort Mackinac, a frontier outpost on Mackinac Island, Michigan. Dr. Beaumont nursed St. Martin back to health, but he was surprised to discover that a gastric fistula had healed open to the skin, which the doctor was unable to close. However, the patient gave his consent for the physician to observe through the fistula rates of digestion and to analyze gastric juices during studies undertaken at Fort Mackinac, at Fort Niagara, New York, and at Fort Crawford, Wisconsin. Valid to this day, Sir William Osler described Beaumont's discoveries in his 1902 essay, "A Backwood Physiologist."

Florence Nightingale (1820-1910), the founder of modern nursing, introduced women nurses in 1854 to care for British soldiers wounded in the Crimean War (1853-1856). In the American Civil War (1861-1865), the United States Sanitary Commission revolutionized the military hospital system to save the lives of the sick and wounded, too often neglected to die of diarrhea and dysentery. Miss Dorthea Dix, Florence Nightingale's American counterpart, recruited nurses to care for Union and Rebel casualties. After the War of the Rebellion, civilian hospitals benefitted from the implementation of those nursing programs and sanitary protocols that protected civilians from the scourge of contagion.

New therapies to prevent malnutrition and to treat infectious disease evolved from wartime experience. Vitamin-C deficiency (scurvy) was prevented, as it had been in the British Navy, when in the winter of 1863, General Joseph Hooker supplemented the Army of Potomac soldiers' rations of salt pork, hard tack, and coffee with fresh vegetables. First available only to the military, Penicillin proved effective in curing staphylococcal and streptococcal infections in American troops during World War II. Ironically, poison gas, used by the Germans against the Allied Troops in World War I, was transformed to HN2 (Nitrogen Mustard), through the research of Leon O. Jacobson, MD, and his co-workers at The University of Chicago, Drs. Guzman Barone, George Kalnitsky, and Michael Bonfiglio, as the first chemotherapeutic agent effective against Hodgkin Lymphoma.

Scientists working on the Manhattan Project produced not only the Atomic Bomb that ended World War II, but made available radioisotopes of Cesium, Cobalt, and Iodine for the radiotherapy of cancer, and other radionuclides for the diagnosis of many diseases by doctors specializing in nuclear medicine. The Space Race of the Cold War (1947-1991) yielded computer technology enabling the development of advanced imaging systems like Computerized Tomography (CT scans), Magnetic Resonance Imaging (MRI), and Positron Emission Tomography (PET scans), which rapidly gained widespread use in civilian medical practice.

TROPICAL MEDICINE

One of the most significant contributions of military medicine came from the conquest of tropical disease. Charles Louis Alphonse Laveran (1845-1922), a French Army surgeon stationed at Constantine, Algeria, first described in 1880, parasites in the blood of a patient with malaria. He received the Nobel Prize in Medicine in 1907 for his discovery. Subsequent studies in the early 20th Century by Sir Patrick Manson and Ronald Ross, a British surgeon in the Indian Army Medical Service, elucidated the life cycle of the malaria parasite. Sir Ronald Ross received the Nobel Prize in 1902 for his demonstration that malaria was transmitted by mosquitoes (anopheles).

Santo Domingo (Haiti) experienced an epidemic of yellow fever in 1493, one year after a visit by Christopher Columbus. In the first months of 1793, three hundred years later, 4041 persons died of yellow fever in Philadelphia. Napoleon's aspirations for a Western Empire in Louisiana were dashed in the early years of the 19th Century (1800-1803) when 20,000 men of General LeClerc's French Army in Haiti were annihilated by yellow fever and by the rebel Francois Dominique Toussaint L'Ouverture (1743?-1803).

After nearly another 100 years, Dr. Carlos J. Finlay (1833-1915), a Cuban physician, convinced members of the U.S. Army Yellow Fever Commission to undertake studies which showed yellow fever was spread by a mosquito (first proclaimed by Dr. Finlay in 1881), later identified as *Aedes aegytpi*. Major Walter Reed, who had demonstrated earlier the modus by which typhoid fever was spread, headed the Yellow Fever Commission, which worked closely with Major William C. Gorgas (1854-1920), Sanitary Chief of Havana, to exterminate mosquitoes in the city. Gorgas and his staff rendered Havana free of yellow fever for the first time in 150 years. The U.S. Army Medical Center in Washington, D.C. was named in honor of Dr. Walter Reed (1851-1902). Suppression of endemic yellow fever by Major Gorgas and the Army later permitted the construction of the Panama Canal.

The Surgeon General of the U.S. Army supported the University of Chicago-Army Medical Research Project, the Malaria Project, at Stateville Penitentiary in Joliet, Illinois. There, from 1944 to 1964, Dr.

Alf Sven Alving (1902-1965) directed the research of army medical officers and inmate volunteers who developed a preventive regimen and cure of *Plasmodium vivax* malaria, a result of their studies of Primaquine, an 8-aminoquinoline. Moreover, they discovered the cause of primaquine-sensitive hemolytic anemia, erythrocyte glucose-6-phosphate dehydrogenase deficiency.

After 1964, during the Vietnam War, under the inspired leadership of Dr. Robin D. Powell (1934-), army medical officers, inmate staff and volunteers on the Malaria Project, developed drug regimens for the prevention and cure of multi-drug resistant *Plasmodium falciparum* malaria prevalent in Southeast Asia and in other parts of the world.

Thus, the application of research findings by Army physicians eliminated the scourge of typhoid fever, yellow fever, and malaria from the United States and many other places in the world.

Appendix Two

Reveal Stateville Revolt by Four 'Black Muslims'

Rebellion among Stateville prison inmates who say they are members of the Black Muslim cult has put three of them in isolation cells and one in the detention hospital for psychiatric examination, Warden Frank J. Pate disclosed yesterday.

Pate said the trouble apparently was an outgrowth of a United States Supreme court decision June 22 in the case of Thomas Cooper, 32, a Black Muslim murderer confined to the segregation division.

Court Orders Inquiry

The high court ruled that lower courts erred in dismissing his suit which claimed his rights were violated by refusal of prison authorities to allow him to practice his religion. The high tribunal ordered the federal District court to investigate Cooper's claim.

Pate said the four rebellious prisoners were confined in the segregation division, where trouble makers are kept. He said each smashed safety glass from a light fixture in his cell and challenged guards to "come on in and get me." The four had been sentenced from Cook county.

The first was Hobson Norris, 33, serving a life term for murder. Guards entered his cell and overpowered him Thursday. He was taken to the detention hospital.

Three Others Named

Two others who revolted Thursday were Gerald Chapman, 25, serving 60 years for rape, and Thomas Washington, 25, serving 2 to 6 years for robbery. Robert Langford, 19, serving 60 years for murder, rebelled yesterday. All three finally left their cells voluntarily.

Several days ago the four and other professed Black Muslims submitted lengthy written demands to the warden, Pate said. He said they asked access to the prison chapel six or seven times a day to pray. Other demands were that they be given a special cook and special food and that they be permitted to distribute Black Muslim literature among fellow prisoners.

The demands were rejected.

CHICAGO TRIBUNE SAT. 4 July 1964

June 1966

Volume 1. Volume 3 is expected later in the year. Purchase may be arranged through the Maruzen Company, Ltd., P.O. Box 605, Tokyo Central, Tokyo, Japan.

The books will make available to the world scientific community much information heretofore published only in the Japanese language. Prepared by 14 renowned Japanese scholars, the three-volume work brings together and summarizes Japanese contributions in the field of parasitology since 1876. It was produced under the direction of the Meguro Parasitological Museum, Tokyo, Japan, and supported in part by a grant from the National Institute of Allergy and Infectious Diseases, one of the nine institutes of the Public Health Service's National Institutes of Health.

A large part of Volume 2 consists of a monograph by Yoshitaka Komiya on the metacercariae found in Japan and adjacent countries. There are many references to papers of metacercariae of trematodes which have been written in Japanese and thus are relatively unfamiliar to European and American parasitologists. The remainder of the volume consists of articles on *Paragonimus* by Ichiro Miyazaki and *Eurytrema* by Itoku Miyata, and a review of the genus *Fasciola* in Japan by Shozo Watanabe.

LEPROSY DRUG TESTED AS AN ANTIMALARIAL

A new use for an old drug is now being tested on several hundred U.S. soldiers in the South Vietnamese highlands. In limited tests in the U.S., the drug—dapsone, which has been considered primarily an antileprosy drug—is said to have protected patients against the resistant strain of *Plasmodium falciparum*. Last year, almost 1,000 GIs were stricken by that strain, which has proved resistant to the chloroquine and primaquine antimalarials regularly taken by Americans in Southeast Asia. A Pentagon spokesman says that two out of three Vietcong prisoners have malaria.

BIBLIOGRAPHY OF TROPICAL MEDICINE

Robert Maxwell & Co. Ltd. of Oxford has issued a Bibliography of Tropical Medicine, No. 42 in the series of Maxwell's International Subject Bibliographies. The listing includes 156 books and technical reports published from 1960 through mid-1965. While the emphasis is on British and American works, much literature from other countries is included. As long as the supply lasts, readers may obtain a free copy of this bibliography by writing to Hans M. Zell, Editor, Robert Maxwell & Co. Ltd., Documentation & Supply Centre, Wynflete Building, 1-8, St. Clements, Oxford, England

MDs Alerted on Malaria Case Rise; Up 100% Over 1965

MDs Alerted To Case Rise In Malaria

Medical News—World Wide Report

ATLANTA, GA.—Practicing physicians and public health officials were alerted to the increasing likelihood that they may encounter cases of malaria by the Communicable Disease Center of the U.S. Public Health Service here. The infections may be caused by drug-resistant forms of Plasmodium falciparum, it noted.

The center said that, with a possibly substantial number of cases still to be reported, the known incidence of malaria cases with onsets in this country during the first 11 months of 1966 was 390—more than double the total 1965 figure.

The cases occurred in 78 civilians and 312 military personnel (including veterans discharged from the armed services in 1965 or 1966). Although the incidence of civilian cases was comparable with that of previous years, the number of military cases with onsets through October 1966 represented a ninefold increase over that of the same period in 1965.

An additional 278 cases were diagnosed in American servicemen overseas who were subsequently transferred to the United States for treatment.

Physicians in private practice are increasingly likely to be consulted by per-

Continued on page 18

Continued from page 1

sons with malaria because the incubation period of the disease can be much longer than international travel itineraries, the Communicable Disease Center pointed out. "These may be servicemen, who are often given prolonged home leave upon their return from overseas duty," as well as recently discharged veterans.

Among the 390 cases with onset in the United States, 386 were "imported," the disease having been acquired elsewhere. "These imported cases enhance the risk of focal re-establishment and transmission of malaria in this country and the subsequent occurrence of introduced cases," the report said, defining an introduced case as one acquired by mosquito transmission contracted from an imported case in an area where malaria is not a regular occurrence.

Among the four cases acquired in the United States, two were suspected of having been introduced. They occurred in two siblings who had never traveled or received blood transfusions but lived in proximity to large numbers of personnel who had returned from malarious regions in Asia.

Because U.S. physicians may lack experience with diagnostic techniques for malaria, the Communicable Disease Center has formulated a guide for preparing malaria blood films. The ideal smear incorporates a thick and a thin film. The thick film, placed at one end of the slide, is made by pressing the slide against

a large globule of blood that forms after a finger is punctured. With a quick circular motion, a film is made the size of a dime. Ordinary newsprint should be barely legible through the wet drop.

Making of Thin Film

The thin film is made by first wiping the finger dry and then gently squeezing a small drop of blood from the puncture onto the middle third of the same slide. Next, the edge of another slide is used to spread this drop in width and length.

The blood film should be kept horizontal and protected from dust and insects while drying. The thick film takes a minimum of six hours to dry at room temperature. The slides before use must be

cleaned with mild detergent, rinsed in warm running water then in distilled water, and dipped in ethyl alcohol, 90 to 95 per cent. They may be stored in 95 per cent alcohol or wiped dry with lintless material for immediate use.

Thick and thin blood smears for confirmation of the diagnosis of malaria should be sent through state health department laboratories to the National Malaria Repository, Parasitology Section, Laboratory Branch, Communicable Disease Center, Atlanta, Ga.

Epidemiologic and therapeutic questions on malaria in the United States should be directed to the Communicable Disease Center's Parasitic Diseases Section (Malaria Surveillance Unit).

11th Case of Transfusion Malaria Reported

Medical News—World Wide Report

ATLANTA, GA. — A new case of blood transfusion-induced malaria is the 11th such case reported since 1957 to the Communicable Disease Center of the U.S. Public Health Service here.

Plasmodium falciparum parasites were found in the blood of a 64-year-old man, according to Drs. Tibor Fodor and Howard B. Shookoff, of the City of New York Department of Health, and Dr. Murray Wittner, of the Albert Einstein College of Medicine. The patient had received blood transfusions during a two-year period prior to malaria onset, for continuous massive bleeding from the renal

pelvis. He did not have a history of self-inoculations and had not traveled outside the United States since he emigrated from Italy in 1913.

The infected blood might have come from a donor who lived in New York City temporarily but who had returned to his native Ghana at the time of the investigation.

The Communicable Disease Center said that of the 10 earlier cases, seven were due to P. malariae, one to P. vivax, one to a mixed infection of P. malariae and P. falciparum, and one to an unknown species. The blood donor was identified in only one instance.

... DEPARTMENT OF HEALTH
... SERVICE PROGRAM
... PHS

P. C

VIA AIR MAIL

The Officer-in-Charge
Malaria Project
Illinois State Penitentiary
Box 1112
Joliet, Illinois

late Morgan W. ~~Davis, and a brother of Richard R. Davis~~
Route 1.

Press Citizen 6/27/64

A PARTY GIVEN WEDNESDAY AFTERNOON. BY MIS
Helen Williams and Mrs. John R. Knott at the latter's hom
715 River street, provided an opportunity for a number of Iov
Citians to meet one of the University of Iowa's most famo
correspondence students, Nathan Leopold.

Mr. and Mrs. Leopold spent a day here en route from the
home in San Juan, Puerto Rico, to Lincoln, Nebr., where M
Leopold is taking part in the annual conference of the Chur
of the Brethren, with which he has been associated since l
release from Stateville penitentiary in Joliet, Ill., six years as
He was to make several addresses at the conference, includi
a major one today.

Nathan Leopold had completed his first year of law at t
University of Chicago when in 1924 he was sentenced to l
for murder and 99 years for kidnaping for his part in the hig
ly publicized Bobby Franks case. In 1930, he wrote to t
University of Iowa to inquire about correspondence work.
personal correspondence with Miss Williams, then head of th
department, has continued since that time.

Meanwhile, Mr. Leopold completed several courses by ma
— at least three in mathematics, one in philosophy and on
in Hebrew literature. He commented Wednesday that th
mathematics work in particular had provided him with th
basis for teaching which he has done recently at the Univer
sity in San Juan.

Mr. Leopold's 99-year term was cut to 85 years by Adlt
Stevenson, then governor of Illinois, after Leopold had serve
as a human guinea pig in malaria experiments in prison dui
ing World War II. He had served more than 33 years in pr
son when his parole was granted in February, 1958.

His autobiographical "Ninety-Nine Years Plus Life", writte
at Stateville, is currently being made into a film by Don Mui
ray, producer of "One Man's Way". Mr. Murray, like M
Leopold, is a member of the Church of the Brethren, whic
has missionary projects all over the world. Approximatel
two-thirds of the movie will be made in Hollywood and th
remainder in Puerto Rico, where the work of the church an
Mr. Leopold's related activity of recent years will be po:
trayed.

Iowa City Press-Citizen 6/27/64

Figure in 1924 Thrill-Killing —

Nathan Leopold Dead

CHICAGO (AP) — Nathan F. Leopold, the brilliant son of a wealthy family who shocked the nation in 1924 when he and a friend murdered a young boy just for a thrill, has died in Puerto Rico, his attorney, reported today.

Attorney Elmer Gertz said Leopold, 66, had died Sunday night at Mimya Hospital in the Santurce section of San Juan. He said death was caused by a heart attack.

Leopold was paroled from an Illinois penitentiary on March 13, 1958, after serving 33 years, six months and two days for the thrill slaying with Richard Loeb of 14-year-old Bobby Franks. Loeb was killed in a fight with another convict in 1936.

When he was released, Leopold went to Puerto Rico as a $10 a month laboratory technician in a missionary hospital. In 1959 he entered the University of Puerto Rico, took a masters degree in social medicine and went to work for the

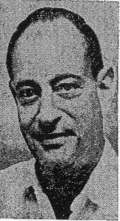

NATHAN LEOPOLD

Puerto Rican health department.

In February 1961 Leopold married Trudy Feld Garcia de Quevedo, the middleaged widow of a San Juan physician. Two years later he was discharged from parole and became a free man.

The Leopold-Loeb case was one of the most sensational of the 1920s and horrified the nation.

The nude body of the Franks boy, a distant relative of Loeb's, was found in a culvert on Chicago's South Side on May 22, 1924. He had been bludgeoned to death.

A pair of eyeglasses nearby led the police to Leopold, then 19 and the son of a vice president of Sears Roebuck. He implicated Loeb, who was 18.

Clarence Darrow, considered the greatest defense lawyer of the time, defended them in a

trial that lasted more than a month.

Darrow had the pair plead guilty so they would be tried before Judge John R. Gaverly without a jury. Then the lawyer fought to save them from execution, bringing forward a string of psychiatrists to testify that the youths were mentally ill but not legally insane. The lawyer closed with a three-day summation denouncing capital punishment.

Two weeks later Judge Gaverly sentenced the pair to life imprisonment for murder and 99 years for kidnaping. He recommended that they never be paroled.

Leopold and Loeb organized the prison correspondence school, and Leopold reorganized the prison library. Early in World War II he was a guinea pig in tests of new drugs for use against malaria. He also studied widely, learning 27 languages and became an authority in several sciences, including ornithology and mathematics.

Gov. Adlai Stevenson in 1949 commuted his 99-year kidnap sentence to 85 years for his work in the malaria tests. This made him eligible for parole in 1953, but it was denied him then and again in 1955 and 1956. Two years later the board turned him loose.

Shortly before release he was asked if he felt he had paid his debt to society.

"Atonement, expiation, that's impossible for me to say," he replied. "I don't know how to measure punishment.

"I have been here 33 years. I have lost all the people near and dear to me—my father, my aunt, an older brother. I have forfeited any chance to make any kind of a success in the world. I have forfeited a chance for a wife and family. Forfeited every chance for any happiness. Now whether that's enough I don't know. Other people will have to decide."

Pastor To Spend Month in Germany

The Rev. W a l t e r J. Olsen, pastor of Faith United Church of Christ, will be in Germany for the month of September on a study exchange tour. He is one of 10 United Church of Christ pastors from the United States participating in the program hosted by the Evangelical Church of the Union in Germany.

In small groups, members of this year's tour will be visiting in parishes in a variety of places of interest with the trip being concluded by participation in an ecumenical conference in Berlin. Pastor Olsen will return to Iowa City Oct. 2.

The Rev. John Moore will preach at Faith United Church Sunday and the Rev. Harold Duerksen will preach on the other Sundays in September.

"KISSING DISEASE"

Infectious mononucleosis, also known as the kissing disease, occurs most often in persons between 10 and 35 years of age, according to Encyclopaedia Britannica.

Thrill-Killer Leopold Dies At Age 66

Leased Wire to The Register

SAN JUAN, PUERTO RICO—Nathan Leopold, who with Richard Loeb shocked the world by kidnaping and murdering 14-year-old Bobby Franks for a thrill in 1924, died a quiet death Sunday evening in a hospital here. He was 66.

He spent the later years of his life in an attempt at atonement and at the end gave his body to science. An official at Mimiya Hospital, where he died of a heart attack, said he had willed his body to the University of Puerto Rico for medical research.

His personal physician, Dr. Ramon Suarez, jr., reported that Leopold urged him shortly before he died to make sure his eyes reached the university's eye bank in time.

Leopold suffered several heart attacks in recent years and was stricken in April with a disease affecting his heart and lungs, according to his Chicago lawyer, Elmer Gertz, who reported Leopold's death.

He had been hospitalized about 10 days before he died, Gertz said.

Life Plus 99 Years

Leopold, of a wealthy Chicago family, was sentenced to life plus 99 years in prison on Sept. 10, 1924, for the killing of Franks, a distant relative of Loeb.

Leopold was 19 years old at that the crime for which he was imprisoned half of his life never was far from his thoughts.

"The crime is definitely still in the central part of my consciousness," he said in an interview earlier this year.

But after 13 years of freedom, Leopold was able to say: "I would say that, on the whole, I have had a good life — even many parts of the prison years. How many people outside prison have time to pursue such purely non-remunerative subjects as Egyptian hieroglyphics and the theory of relativity? I did."

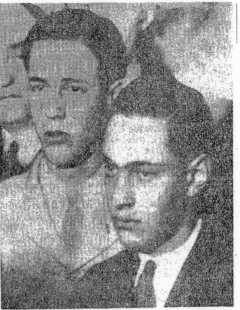

WIREPHOTO (AP)

At Leopold Trial

Richard Loeb (left) and Nathan Leopold are pictured at the time of their 1924 murder trial. Leopold died Sunday evening in his Puerto Rico home. Loeb was killed in prison in 1936.

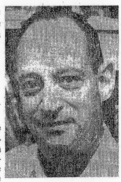

Wirephoto (AP)

Nathan Leopold
Willed Body to Science

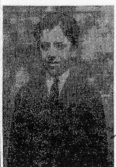

Bibliography

Baatz, Simon: *For the Thrill of It, Leopold, Loeb, and the Murder that Shocked Chicago*; HarperCollins, New York, 2008, pp.541.

DeGowin, Elmer L. & DeGowin, Richard L.: *Bedside Diagnostic Examination*, (3rd edition), Macmillan Publishing Co., New York, 1976, pp. 952.

Gordon-Reed, Annette: *The Hemingses of Monticello*; W.W. Norton & Co., New York, 2008, pp. 798.

Isenberg, Nancy: *Fallen Founder, The Life of Aaron Burr;* Viking-Penguin, New York, 2007, pp. 540.

Kantrowitz, Nathan: *Close Control, Managing a Maximum Security Prison, The Story of Ragen's Stateville Penitentiary*; Harrow & Heston, New York, 1996, pp. 217.

Masterson, Karen M.: *The Malaria Project, The U.S. Government's Secret Mission to Find a Miracle Cure*; New American Library, New York, 2014, pp. 405.

Spillane, Joseph P.: *Coxsackie, The Life and Death of Prison Reform*, Johns Hopkins University Press, Baltimore, 2014, pp. 296.

Book Two:
Discovery is Our Business
Stories of Doctors Who Made
Discovery Their Business

CONTENTS—BOOK II: DISCOVERY IS OUR BUSINESS

Preface... 181

Stagg Field... 183

    Enrico Fermi, PhD... 185

    Leon O. Jacobson, MD... 189

    Clifford W. Gurney, MD.. 201

    Sanford B. Krantz, MD.. 211

    William E. Adams, MD.. 214

    Janet D. Rowley, MD... 222

    Henry T. Ricketts, MD.. 225

    Ernest Beutler, MD.. 231

    Kenneth M. Brinkhaus, MD....................................... 235

    Charles B. Huggins, MD.. 241

Acknowledgments... 247

Appendix.. 249

Bibliography... 250

About the Author.. 251

Preface

I imagine reporters from the *Chicago Tribune* smiled, as I did, when they read the plaque above the door to the laboratory of Dr. Charles B. Huggins: ***Discovery is Our Business***. They had come to The University of Chicago to interview Dr. Huggins when they learned the committee in Stockholm had just announced that Dr. Huggins would receive the 1966 Nobel Prize in Medicine, shared with Dr. Peyton Rous of the Rockefeller Institute.

In recalling this event that happened over 50 years ago, it occurred to me that if I hadn't realized it when I was associated with the School of Medicine for over a decade as a medical student, resident, research associate, and assistant professor, The University of Chicago was an extraordinary place where good people made good things happen. I had the unusual privilege of working with remarkable doctors, who, in addition to teaching medical students, and caring for their patients, studied their patients' diseases, and found new ways of treating their illnesses, even curing them.

In addition to training physicians to practice in their communities, a mission of The University of Chicago School of Medicine was to prepare graduates for careers in academic medicine. I recall being told that 15% of Chicago graduates entered academic medicine, third in the nation behind Harvard and Hopkins. Accordingly, my classmates and I had the opportunity to pursue research projects in medical school and during residency training, supervised by members of a full-time faculty. The success of this mission occurred to me when I reflected on the number of friends in my class of 1959—over 20% of my classmates—who selected careers in academic medicine. Moreover, I can recall at least 10 colleagues on the faculty in The

University of Iowa College of Medicine who had graduated from The University of Chicago over the years.

Drs. William E. Adams and Kenneth M. Brinkhous, whose stories I tell, grew up in rural Iowa. Both graduated from The University of Iowa College of Medicine. Dr. Adams joined the surgical faculty at The University of Chicago, and Dr. Brinkhous joined the faculty of The University of North Carolina as Chief of the Department of Pathology and Laboratory Medicine. Both men served as leaders of their specialty associations in America, and both were recognized internationally as leaders in their fields of specialty because of their discoveries that helped patients return to healthier lives.

The reader met my chief, Dr. Jacobson, and my mentor, Dr. Clifford Gurney, in Book I, in which I detailed my experiences in the Army from 1963 to 1965. I joined them, and other former teachers, later colleagues and friends, on the faculty of The University of Chicago from 1965, and after my service to 1968, and report in Book II about their remarkable achievements. So Book II is a natural sequel to Book I.

If the narratives of these doctor-scientists inspire a medical student or graduate—the stories of my medical heroes—who inspired me, will prove worth telling.

Stagg Field

A persistent dismal drizzle drenched the banner, demanding in big black letters: "End the War in Vietnam." Students had hung their mandate between the gargoyle downspouts under the fourth floor widows of Abbott Hall, facing north to Stagg Field.

Sandy Krantz and I were here on this chilly winter Saturday, 2 December 1967, to witness the dedication of the site where the squash courts had been in the West Stands of Stagg Field, the stands torn down years ago.

We had come, not to celebrate the glory days of football—they were glory days, indeed—when The University of Chicago (U. of C.), a founding member of the Big 10 Conference from 1896-1939, won seven Big 10 titles from 1899 to 1924, and national championships in 1905 and in 1913. That was when legendary coach, Amos Alonzo Stagg coached student Jay Berwanger, a native of Dubuque, Iowa, to win, in 1935, the first Heisman Trophy. Jay Berwanger turned down invitations to play in the NFL for the Chicago Bears and returned to Iowa where he engaged in a lucrative career manufacturing plastic parts for automobiles. Before the award gained great respect, Jay's Aunt Gussie used his bronze trophy as a doorstop. Now it resides safely in a museum.

Sandy and I joined others, huddled in our overcoats under an open-sided maroon (colors of the U. of C.) canvas tent to commemorate the site where 25 years earlier Chicago Pile #1 (CP-1) went critical in the first self-sustaining atomic chain reaction, initiating the Atomic Age. Standing with scientists, army officers, and others under an adjacent tent, was the 1951 Nobel Laureate in Chemistry, now Head of the U.S. Atomic Energy Commission, Glen Seaborg. He was there with the survivors of that historic day on 2 December

1942 who witnessed—from the balcony of the squash courts in the West Stands—the moment when CP-1 went critical.

The successful outcome of this physics experiment enabled the United States to take the lead in controlling nuclear energy during World War II, denying the Nazis the ability to conquer the world with atomic bombs. But in 2020, Iran, a Middle Eastern sponsor of world terrorism, races to build an atomic bomb, and Kim Jong Un of North Korea threatens Asia with ballistic missiles capable of carrying bombs with a range as far as California. The concept of Mutual Assured Destruction (MAD) during the Cold War, embraced by Russia and the U.S., meant we survived the era without a nuclear war. Will current residents of the planet realize, or care, about the prospects of such a devastating future?

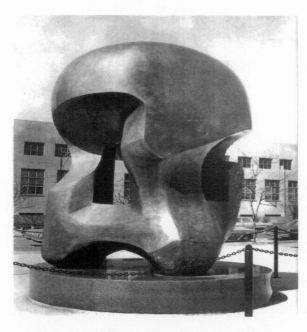

NUCLEAR ENERGY
BY HENRY MOORE

Enrico Fermi, PhD

Dr. Herbert Anderson, Fermi's graduate student in 1942, now the Director of the Fermi Institute for Nuclear Studies, in the building across the street, took the microphone of the public address system to describe the momentous event in which he participated 25 years ago.

As I remember Dr. Anderson's words, he said something like this:

"The physicists, Army officers, and representatives from industry—some of you are here today—stood on the balcony of the squash court looking at the atomic pile (CP-1), fifty-seven layers of pure graphite blocks, enclosing and moderating the neutron flux from inserted cubes of Uranium-235 (U-235). I stood on the balcony, axe in hand ready to sever a rope. One end of the rope was tied to the balcony rail in front of me. The other end ran through a pulley in the ceiling to suspend a cadmium control rod, poised to drop into the pile and shut down an atomic chain reaction should it get out of control, explode, and obliterate CHICAGO's SOUTH SIDE."

"Dr. Fermi, after making calculations using his slide rule, ordered George Weil, standing on the floor of the squash court, to pull out, a few centimeters, the main cadmium control rod that absorbed neutrons, controlling the reaction. Immediately, the neutron scalers started clicking faster, indicating the increased release of neutrons. Repeating the sequence, the faster clicking of the scalers raised tension in the observers. Just when the rapid clicking of the neutron scalers sounded like something might happen, Fermi said, 'I'm hungry. Let's go to lunch.' And we did."

"When the group returned to the squash court after lunch, Fermi resumed his calculations. The main cadmium control rod was progressively withdrawn, accompanied by accelerated clicking of the neutron scalers until Fermi said, 'The pile has gone critical! Reinsert the control rod.'"

Resting on the site of the squash court before us, *Nuclear Energy*— the nine-foot high statue executed by the famous sculptor, Henry Moore—was hidden from our view by a maroon canvas shroud, soaked with rain. At 2:00 pm, 2 December 1942, on the campus of The University of Chicago, the first self-sustaining nuclear chain reaction initiated the Atomic Age. And now, at 2:00 pm, Saturday, 2 December 1967, exactly 25 years after CP-1 went critical, Laura Fermi, the widow of Enrico Fermi, stepped forward, grasped a rope attached to the canvas shroud to unveil the huge sculpture. The rope broke! Henry Moore joined Laura Fermi as they both grasped another rope to pull the wet canvas from the monument. With effort, the two unveiled Henry Moore's *Nuclear Energy*. Observers gasped. Some said the massive black obsidian statue, glistening in the drizzle, looked like the mushroom cloud of an atomic bomb blast. Others said it was a black death's head (skull). Some said it resembled a cathedral, while others said it looked like a football helmet.

THE MET LAB

The Metallurgical Laboratory (The Met Lab) was the code name at The University of Chicago where Enrico Fermi and his staff worked on the Manhattan Project during World War II. Their demonstration that an atomic chain reaction could be controlled enabled General Leslie R. Groves, the Director of the Manhattan Project, to build up three cities: Oak Ridge, Tennessee, to produce Uranium-235; Hanford, Washington, to produce Plutonium; and Los Alamos, New Mexico, to make atomic bombs—a tremendous industrial undertaking, all done in secrecy.

If the United States Military was forced to invade the Japanese Islands, where all citizens were ready to fight to their death, Army Officers projected one-half to a million American boys would lose their lives. My future father-in-law, a Master Sergeant, serving in the South Pacific, was one of those men scheduled to be deployed for the invasion. It was estimated more than two million Japanese would die fighting for their homeland, and the war would last until late 1946. The Japanese warlords refused to surrender—even after General Curtis LeMay's Air Force fire-bombed Tokyo—when they were warned of the devastation to be wrought by atomic bombs.

Ordered by President Harry S. Truman, Colonel Paul W. Tibbets flew the B-29, *Enola Gay* (named for his mother) from Tinian and dropped *Little Boy*, a Uranium bomb, on Hiroshima on 6 August 1945. It obliterated this military-industrial Japanese city, killing 140,000 residents. The Japanese still refused to surrender. On 9 August 1945, the B-29 named *Bock's Car*, dropped *Fat Man*, a Plutonium implosion bomb on Nagasaki, killing 70,000 persons, showing that the

U.S. had more than one atomic bomb and the determination to use them. General Douglas MacArthur, who knew the Oriental mind from his long service in the Philippines, told his physician, Dr. Roger O. Egeberg, the Japanese would view the atomic blasts as something supernatural and let the Emperor save face, and surrender. He did.

The horror of the bombs' destruction led to the concept of Mutual Assured Destruction (MAD) for 45 years during the Cold War to the present, when atomic bombs have never been used in warfare. Instead, people the world over have benefitted from the peaceful use of atomic energy from the generation of electricity to medical and other civilian uses.

The Medical Advisor to the Metallurgical Laboratory, a 31-year old second year Resident in Internal Medicine, Leon O. Jacobson, MD, was appointed as the Health Officer for the persons working on the Manhattan Project. It was Dr. Jacobson's job to physically examine the scientists, and to monitor the blood counts of Enrico Fermi, Herbert Anderson, and other members of the group to ensure they were not exposed to toxic levels of radiation in their work with U-235 and other radioisotopes. He was selected because of his interest and research on the effects of radiation on the sensitive blood-producing cells in the bone marrow. Nurse Edna K. Marks and Evelyn Gaston worked in the special clinic he set up to care for the scientists, and later, worked in his research laboratory for the years until they retired. After World War II, Dr. Enrico Fermi, the 1938 Nobel Laureate in Physics, served on the faculty of The University of Chicago until he died at age 53 on 28 November1954. His physicist colleagues in Italy had given him the nickname, *The Pope of Physics*, because, they said, he was never wrong. Chicago survived intact, because his slide rule calculations on 2 December 1942 were never wrong.

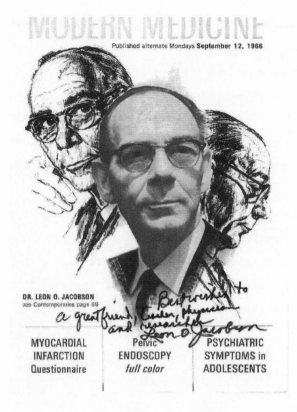

MODERN MEDICINE

Published alternate Mondays **September 12, 1966**

DR. LEON O. JACOBSON
see Contemporaries page 99

Best wishes to a great friend, teacher, physician and researcher

Leon O. Jacobson

MYOCARDIAL	Pelvic	PSYCHIATRIC
INFARCTION	ENDOSCOPY	SYMPTOMS in
Questionnaire	*full color*	ADOLESCENTS

Leon O. Jacobson, MD

CHEMOTHERAPY OF CANCER

My high school classmate, Tom Ewers, joined me working as common labor on a street paving crew in Iowa City during the summer of 1955 when I was home on vacation from the University of Michigan. In August, Tom invited me to celebrate his 21st birthday by joining him in having a beer in every one of the ten bars in Iowa City. Having consumed small glasses of 3.2% draft beer over the afternoon and evening, we ended our odyssey in the Oasis Bar, fairly sober and good friends. Shortly thereafter, I left for my freshman year of medical school at The University of Chicago, and Tom graduated from The University of Iowa in May 1956, with a degree in education and a diagnosis of Hodgkin lymphoma. He lived four years, the median survival for Hodgkin lymphoma then.

In 1963, as a resident, I saw one of Dr. Jacobson's patients while working in the clinic. In his chart, I read he had received injections of *Compound X* (code name for nitrogen mustard) every month in 1943 for a diagnosis of Hodgkin lymphoma. After the war, his remission of 20 years was sustained by receiving periodic injections of nitrogen mustard.

Clarence Lushbaugh, PhD '42, MD '48, and his coworkers in the Toxicity Lab at U. of C., investigated ways to neutralize agents used in chemical warfare, like mustard gas. They were concerned the Nazis might use it on the battlefield. As Medical Advisor to the lab, Dr. Jacobson knew of Dr. Lushbaugh's research in which he demonstrated the atrophy of lymph nodes and splenic tissue in laboratory rats injected with nitrogen mustard. Together they calculated, on the basis of Dr. Lushbaugh's studies, what they believed to be a non-lethal dose of nitrogen mustard.

With permission from his chief and the patient to conduct a clinical trial in a person for whom all previous treatments had failed, in March 1943, Dr. Jacobson administered nitrogen mustard to a patient with lymphatic leukemia, who had a high white blood cell count and enlarged lymph nodes. After receiving the intravenous infusion, the patient vomited for several hours. Then he recovered, as Dr. Jacobson sat up with the patient for the next 24 hours. The patient's white blood cell count came down and his lymph nodes decreased. He had a remission, which encouraged Dr. Jacobson to treat a patient with Hodgkin lymphoma, whose enlarged lymph nodes diminished in size as the patient went into remission. The patient returned to work and lived for many years thereafter. Dr. Jacobson and his colleagues treated 59 patients with nitrogen mustard (HN2), with the same success in achieving significant remissions. Later studies by other investigators demonstrated that by incorporating HN2 into a multi-drug regimen—Mustargen, Oncovin, Procarbazine, Prednisone , (MOPP)—patients with Hodgkin lymphoma could be cured. In effect, Dr. Jacobson developed the first effective chemotherapy for the treatment of cancer. I wish friend Tom could have benefitted from Dr. Jacobson's work.

SPLEEN SHIELDING

Dr. Eric Simmons, a research associate of Dr. Jacobson's, introduced me to Dr. Clarence Lushbaugh when we visited his laboratory in the Atomic Energy Commission facility in Oak Ridge, Tennessee, where he worked after leaving the U. of C. We had come to Oak Ridge to attend the 10th Annual Meeting of the Bone Marrow Conference. It grew from its first meeting of scientists in Dr. Jacobson's hotel room during a spring meeting of the Federated Scientific Societies in Atlantic City. Later, it became the International Society for Experimental Hematology.

The only paper I remember was given by E. Donnall Thomas, MD, of Cooperstown, New York, in which he reported upon the transplantation of bone marrow cells in dogs. Don Thomas later moved to the University of Washington. He received the 1990 Nobel Prize in Medicine for his successful transplantation of bone marrow cells in patients. As a visiting speaker at The University of Chicago, Dr. Thomas acknowledged Dr. Jacobson's early studies as the basis for his work on bone marrow transplantation in his patients with leukemia and other lethal diseases.

After the war, in the late 1940's, Dr. Jacobson (known by his friends as 'Jake') and his research associates, studied the effects of radiation on the cells of the bone marrow in a program supported by the Atomic Energy Commission for the peaceful use of nuclear energy—*From Swords to Plowshares*. When the investigators infused strontium-89 (Sr-89) into the blood of laboratory mice, it deposited in bone, like calcium did. The radiation emitted from Sr-89 in the bone marrow killed the very radiosensitive blood producing cells, the stem cells, but the mice survived, and they did not become anemic. On further study, Jake and his coworkers saw the spleen had undergone hyperplasia, producing blood cells to compensate for the bone marrow failure. The spleen is an early source of blood production in the human fetus as it is in the mice.

Jake and his team asked the question, "If we exteriorize the spleen on its vascular pedicle, place it in a lead box to protect it from radiation, and then administer a lethal dose of x-rays to the exposed body of the mouse, will it survive?" They did, and it did. The mice survived even if the vascular pedicle was severed only fifteen minutes after the body of the mouse received the dose of radiation. Subsequent experiments, in which minute portions of spleen, or even spleen cells, were infused intravenously after total body irradiation, saved the mice.

Jake concluded, wrongly, that a hormone from the spleen cells facilitated the post-irradiation bone marrow repopulation. However, a research group at Harwell, in England, and Dr. Egon Lorenz, and his associate, Delta Uphoff, at the National Cancer Institute, showed that marked cells in the blood stream repopulated the bone marrow after the radiation. But Jake's early research with the injection of spleen cells prompted these later studies that elucidated the true mechanism leading to survival. Initially, bone marrow cells were harvested by aspirating marrow from the pelvic bones of donors, but with refinement of apheresis technology, enough of the hemopoietic stem cells are harvested from donor peripheral blood for successful transplantation. As a result of many doctors' work, bone marrow transplantation has saved the lives of patients with cancer and genetically related blood diseases.

ERYTHROPOIETIN

They said Lance Armstrong had been "blood doping"—he was accused of receiving infusions of erythropoietin to increase the oxygen-carrying capacity of his red blood cell mass—to give him a competitive edge in winning the *Tour de France* bicycle race. Many heard about erythropoietin in the news, but my introduction to the hormone began a half century before the sports scandal.

I was working as an orderly with nurses on C-54, a surgical ward in The University of Iowa Hospitals and Clinics (UIHC), living at home on vacation, having survived my freshman year in medical school at The University of Chicago. That year, 1956, was a memorable year, not only because I learned a lot about taking care of patients on a busy surgical service, but it was the summer I met my bride-to-be—our marriage lasting almost 60 years.

My father was the Founding Director of the blood bank in UIHC, named after his death, *The Elmer L. DeGowin Memorial Blood Center.* Dr. Lindon Seed, a Chicago surgeon and former director of the nation's first blood bank at Cook County Hospital, told me in a telephone call after my father died, that the Iowa blood center was the oldest *continuously* operating blood bank in the United States. One evening, when both my father and I were home from the hospital, I asked him, "How does the body replenish a pint of blood the donor gives at the blood bank?" He replied, like the professor he was, "When you return to school, ask Dr. Jacobson that question. Jake and his research team are studying that very question."

Indeed, Dr. Jacobson's research group answered my question—erythropoietin. Their studies with experimental animals showed that erythropoietin, which induced primitive bone marrow cells to make red blood cells—when the oxygen-carrying capacity of the blood was reduced by loss of red cells or by hypoxia in the atmosphere—was released into the blood stream from the kidney, its main source of production. They published the results of their research as: Fried, W., Plzak, L.F., Jacobson, L.O., and Goldwasser, E.: *Studies on erythropoiesis III. Factors controlling erythrocyte production*. Proc. Soc. Exper. Biol. & Med. 94: 237-241, 1957. Wally Fried and Lou Plzak were senior medical students. Later, Wally, as a hematologist, pursued his research interest in blood production and became Associate Dean of Rush Medical School in Chicago. Lou Plzak became a Professor of Surgery at Jefferson Medical College in Philadelphia.

You might ask, "How did their research help patients?" Their discovery of the kidney as the source of erythropoietin production explained the poor response to anemia in patients with chronic renal failure, whose waste products were removed from the blood by renal dialysis—compensating for the *exocrine* failure of the kidneys but not for its *endocrine* failure (erythropoietin), requiring blood transfusions to correct the decreased red cell mass. After 25 years of persistent work, the research group of Gene Goldwasser purified erythropoietin, so the gene for the hormone could be cloned to permit Amgen, a fledgling biotech firm in Thousand Oaks, California, to produce recombinant erythropoietin. Administration of recombinant erythropoietin to patients with chronic renal failure meant their physicians no longer had to rely upon blood transfusions to maintain the patients' red blood cell mass. This is hormone replacement therapy. Erythropoietin is to chronic renal failure like insulin is to diabetes. Incidentally, Amgen became the largest biotech firm in the world.

Leon Oris Jacobson was born on 16 December 1911 in Sims, North Dakota, a town so small, his brother bought it, incorporating it in his ranch. Jake's parents, Rachel and John Jacobson, came to North Dakota from Norway. In America, they raised seven children—Jake, his sister and his five brothers—in a strict but loving rural household. Both English and Norwegian were spoken in the home. Jake was delighted when I brought him a copy of the *Decorah Posten*—the only newspaper published in the Norwegian language in the United States. I bought the paper in my wife Karen's hometown, Decorah, Iowa—a hotbed of Norwegians, host at one time to King Olaf of Norway and later to President Barack Obama. It was also the home of the Norwegian-American Museum, and of Luther College.

Jake attended a one-room country school in Sims as the only member of his seventh grade. In nearby Almont High School, he benefitted from teachers who encouraged him to excel in English and mathematics. After attending North Dakota Agricultural College in Fargo for three years, he obtained a job as a teacher in a two-room country school. He returned to college, graduating with a Bachelor of Science Degree. At the suggestion of several of his teachers, Chicago alumni, he decided to apply to medical school at The University of Chicago.

With a Leopold Schepp Foundation Scholarship, and a loan from Shreve Archer of Minneapolis (Archer, Daniels, Midland Corporation—ADM), Jake enrolled as a freshman medical student at Chicago in 1935. After he graduated in 1939, he wrote Archer he planned to intern at Chicago, and Archer forgave his loan. Jake completed internship and residency training in Internal Medicine in The University of Chicago Hospitals and Clinics (UCHC) during World War II, serving as a medical advisor in both the Toxicity Laboratory and in the Metallurgical Laboratory, because of his special interest in hematology. In 1945, he was named head of the Hematology Section in the Department of Medicine after the war.

I remember a lecture Jake gave to my medical classmates. He said there were no curative regimens for patients with lethal hematologic diseases, like leukemia and lymphoma, but there are none for patients with diabetes, either. In both cases, however, physicians help improve their patients' lives. His remarks made an impression on my friends and on me, because of all the specialties in medicine, five of us in the class of 1959, became hematologists: Steven A. Armentrout, James K. Dahl, Richard L. DeGowin, J. David Heywood, and Sanford B. Krantz.

Jake assembled in the Section of Hematology, a remarkable group of persons on the second floor of Argonne Cancer Research Hospital (ACRH), where we had our laboratories. Clifford W. Gurney, my mentor, became head of Hematology when Jake became Chairman of Medicine. Cliff left Chicago to serve as the first Chairman of Medicine at Rutgers Medical School, then Chief of Medicine at Kansas University Medical School. Later, he returned to Chicago as Associate Dean for Clinical Studies; Richard K. Blaisdell was appointed Chairman of Medicine at the University of Hawaii Medical School; Alvin R. Tarlov, became Chief of Medicine at Chicago, then Head of the Henry Kaiser Foundation; Ernest Beutler named Chairman of Medicine City of Hope National Medical Center, Duarte, California; Sanford B. Krantz became Head of Hematology at Vanderbilt Medical School; Robert Weiler, became Director of Hematology at the Lovelace Clinic at the University of New Mexico.

Argonne Cancer Research Hospital (ACRH)
When it opened in 1953, with an annual multimillion dollar budget, supported by the United States Atomic Energy Commission, Dr.

Leon Jacobson was the Founding Director of the Argonne Cancer Research Hospital. His mission was to explore, with his colleagues, the medical use of nuclear energy in the diagnosis and treatment of patients with cancer.

The two underground stories of ACRH contained three state-of-the-art machines to study the potential effectiveness of radiotherapy: a linear accelerator, a Cobalt source, and a Van der Graff generator. Radioisotopes for diagnosis and therapy were prepared in an isotope pharmacy. A conference room, administrative offices, and a sophisticated machine and electronics shop for the fabrication of customized research instruments occupied the first floor. Jake's office and laboratory, and the research laboratories and offices of his colleagues—the members of the Section of Hematology—were on the second floor of ACRH. Patients participating in research studies were admitted to private rooms, at no charge, on the third and fourth floors. Margot Doyle's editorial office and more research laboratories were on the fifth floor. A small animal unit for experimental mice and rats shared the sixth floor with a diagnostic and therapeutic x-ray facility, run by James Bland.

In 1961, when I was a resident, Dr. Jacobson was appointed Chairman of the Department of Internal Medicine. He presided over Grand Rounds in P-117, enlivening the presentations. As an interlocutor, he joked with his colleagues in the audience, requesting comments about the talks—a school teacher calling on his pupils to recite.

It must have been a warm day in 1965. I felt a little guilty leaving the hospital after putting in only a ten-hour day, but I had seen my patients, and I had completed the next step in the experiment in my lab on the second floor of ACRH. Moreover, I knew Karen was parked at the curb at 6:00 pm on Ellis Avenue outside the rear entrance to the ACRH waiting to take us home.

If I felt guilty about leaving early, the feeling was compounded when I realized the lanky man standing on the grass, his long arms draped on the roof of my car, talking to my wife, was my boss, Dr. Jacobson, Director of the ACRH, Chairman of Internal Medicine— the person responsible for my academic appointment, my salary, and my research funding. When I approached the car, he greeted me, turned and walked down the sidewalk on his way home.

Seated in the car, I asked Karen, "What were you talking about?" She said, "I congratulated him on being named Dean of The Division of Biological Sciences and the School of Medicine.

And he said, 'I hope I don't screw up.'"

I first met Dr. Jacobson in 1958. It was during my junior clerkship, assigned to the Hematology Service, when my attending physician asked me to tell Dr. Jacobson about one of his patients hospitalized on our service. The receptionist in the Hematology Clinic Dr. Jacobson attended that morning said he was in one of the examining rooms with his patient and would be returning to the conference room in a few minutes where I could talk to him. How would this internationally famous doctor and scientist respond to me, a lowly medical student, I wondered nervously? I need not have worried, because shortly thereafter, he stepped into the inner corridor of the clinic, his arms over the shoulders of senior medical students—one on each side of him—talking and smiling. Jake loved to care for his patients and teach medical students and residents.

The last time I saw Jake was in April 1992. I was one of the invited speakers at a two-day scientific symposium for Dr. Jacobson. It recognized his eightieth birthday, the year before, and occurred during the year-long series of ceremonies celebrating the centennial of the founding of The University of Chicago. Jake's colleagues in research, his friends on the faculty, and former students gathered in the hospital auditorium, P-117, to present research papers in his honor. I shared the podium with a remarkable group of people: Clifford Gurney, Sandy Krantz, Wally Fried, Janet Rowley, and other scientists who had worked with Jake. We were introduced by Jake's long-time research collaborator, and his biographer, Eugene Goldwasser.

After the morning session of the first day, Wally Fried and I had lunch with Jake. I remember Wally asked him how he had arrived at a safe dose of HN2 that led to remissions in patients with Hodgkin lymphoma who had received the nitrogen mustard infusion during the first clinical trial. Jake replied that he depended upon calculations made from the results of Clarence Lushbaugh's studies with experimental rats.

Karen, son Bobby, and I left Chicago in 1968, after I had been associated, one way or another, with the U. of C. for 13 years. Karen had worked as Orthoptist in the Eye Clinic in UCHC for Dr. Frank Newell with Receptionist Lois Owen and with Nurse Jeff Posten, both of whom became our life-long friends. At the time of the symposium, I was Professor of Medicine and Hematology and the Founding Director of The University of Iowa Cancer Center. Karen and I had checked into the Palmer House downtown planning to see Lois and our other friends after the symposium.

On 14 April 1992, during a break in the symposium, I received a message from Lois Owen that construction workers had mistakenly breached the wall preventing the Chicago River from entering the tunnel system supplying electrical facilities for the buildings downtown, resulting in a flood and a total blackout. Karen had planned to join me for a dinner honoring Jake at the Smart Museum on campus, but I had no way of knowing in this pre-cell phone era, where she was. Later, at the museum, I was talking to Cliff Gurney, my mentor, anxiously awaiting Karen's arrival when she walked in the door.

Elated to see her, we embraced, and I told her how glad I was to see her safe. With a twinkle in his eye, Cliff said, "That's odd. Dick seemed more concerned about whether his slides for tomorrow's talk were safe." Thanks a lot, Cliff.

Karen had taken a taxi from the Planetarium to the Palmer House to find that it was totally dark. The cabbie warned her not to go in there, but she found an accommodating Bell Hop, who escorted her with his flashlight up seven flights of dark stairs to our room. He waited while she packed, then guided her downstairs where she took a cab to the Conrad Hilton on Michigan Avenue. South of the flood, it had retained electrical power.

We were fortunate to see Jake that April, because he died later in the year on 20 September 1992. Framed on the wall of my den is the cover of the 12 September 1966 issue of *Modern Medicine*, featuring Jake's portrait in triplicate, inscribed, "Best wishes to a great friend, teacher, physician and researcher. Leon O. Jacobson." Written boldly in his beautiful Palmer-method cursive script, it is characteristic of a school teacher and friend I hold in high esteem. I am sure it is obvious to you, as it is to me, the kind words in the inscription tell more about the scribe than their recipient.

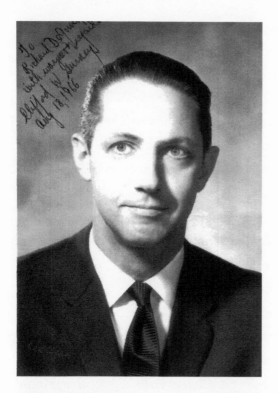

Clifford W. Gurney, MD

Where did I first learn of stem cells? I am not sure, but it must have been in the Histology Course during the first year of medical school, taught by Dr. William Bloom, coauthor of our textbook of histology by Maximow and Bloom. Alexander Maximow concluded in 1909, from his study of bone marrow cells in tissue culture, that the primitive cell that gave rise to precursors of white cells, red cells and platelets, resembled a small lymphocyte. To my knowledge, no one had confirmed his theory with their own independent studies, and when I asked, nobody could identify the hemopoietic (blood producing) stem cell on a bone marrow smear for me.

My next serious thoughts about stem cells came during a great elective course I took during my second year, *Granulomas and Tumors,* taught by a superb teacher, Paul E. Steiner, MD, PhD. He looked like a real professor, slender, straight posture, small mustache, gray suit and vest—his Phi Beta Kappa key dangling from a gold watch chain. If a scribe took down, word-for-word, his clear, logical, and interesting lectures, they could have been published without a need for change. With an interest in Civil War history, I treasure a copy of his book, *Medical-Military Portraits of Union and Confederate Generals.*

I heard about leukemia from Dr. Steiner's guest hematologist, Richard K. Blaisdell, MD, an outstanding young clinician, who later became Chairman, Department of Medicine, The University of Hawaii. He had a masterful grasp of the literature, surprising me by citing the work—which elucidated a hemolytic mechanism in the blood of patients with pernicious anemia—by the research group at The University of Iowa, led by Dr. Elmer DeGowin.

Dr. Steiner's young assistant was Werner Kirsten, MD, a brilliant pathologist, after whom the Kirsten Virus that caused Mouse Leukemia was named, and who would later become Chairman of Pathology at The University of Chicago. The discussions by these two brilliant men of the clinical and pathologic aspects of the diseases—while we examined slides from patients with those illnesses under our microscopes—were outstanding, talking extemporaneously, as they walked the aisles between our classroom tables. I worked hard, and I enjoyed the course—especially when I learned that Dr. Steiner had given me an A+ for the course.

My colleague, Dr. Charles E. Platz, former Director of Surgical Pathology at the University of Iowa Hospitals and Clinics, began as a freshman medical student at U. of C., working for the next four years as a research assistant in Dr. Kirsten's laboratory. He cared for a group of rats infected with the Kirsten virus by neonatal injection of mouse leukemic cells. At the conclusion of the experiment—after which the rats would normally be sacrificed—he continued to care for them for another twelve weeks to discover they had developed solid tumors; i.e., sarcomas.

Learning about leukemia led me to think that if I could study the controls that induced the stem cell to differentiate into its specialized descendants—white cells, red cells, platelets, and lymphocytes—and still reproduce itself, maybe I could uncover the pathologic mechanisms involved in leukemia and intervene to find a cure. So, anticipating an elective quarter of research as a resident in Internal Medicine, I asked Dr. Jacobson, if anyone in his Section of Hematology was doing research on stem cells. He replied, "See Gurney. He just returned from a year's sabbatical in England at Oxford, studying stem cells with Dr. Laszlo Lajtha."

After I introduced myself to Cliff Gurney and requested his help with a research project, his warm handshake immediately put me at ease. Little did I know then he would become my mentor, hire me for my first job in academic medicine, and seal a friendship lasting fifty-three years—until the day he died on 10 April 2014, one day before his 90th birthday.

When I told him I wanted to find out how the replication and differentiation of hemopoietic stem cells were controlled in health and disease, he said, "Of course. That is our ultimate goal. But first, let's start with a straight forward question, work that needs to be done and will result in a publication. I will tell Diana Hoffstra, my research assistant, to expect you in the lab this afternoon, where you can begin to develop a dose-response curve for a bioassay of erythropoietin." What remarkably good advice, considering my research electives as a medical student had failed to result in a contribution to the medical literature.

At first, scientists thought red blood cell production was increased when the bone marrow itself became hypoxic. Residents living in the mountains—at high altitudes with diminished atmospheric oxygen—had elevated hematocrits, indicating an increased red blood cell mass. In 1906, Carnot and Deflandre proposed that a hormone was released into the blood of anemic patients to stimulate the bone marrow to make blood, rather than the bone marrow's direct response to hypoxia.

The Bioassay

The lack of a sensitive assay for the hormone delayed understanding of the mechanisms involved until the 1943 Nobel Laureate in Chemistry, George de Hevesy, showed how radioactive iron ($59Fe$), was incorporated into the hemoglobin of newly formed red blood cells. This meant an investigator could accurately quantitate erythropoiesis (red blood cell production).

Injecting plasma containing elevated levels of erythropoietin from an anemic subject into a rat or mouse might increase red blood cell production in the recipient, but the rodent's own erythropoiesis provided too much "background noise" to show a difference. Therefore, to suppress the assay animal's erythropoiesis, so a difference could be observed between the activity in the assay sample and the recipient's ongoing erythropoiesis, investigators fed rats only water for 36 hours, which curtailed red blood cell production (the starved rat bioassay), or they transfused mice with red blood cells to achieve hematocrits of 75% (normal 45%) shutting down blood production (the plethoric mouse bioassay). In a series of studies, Cliff Gurney showed that the incorporation of $59Fe$ into the red cells of the plethoric mouse, proved to be the most sensitive bioassay for erythropoietin.

His bioassay of the fluid containing high levels of erythropoietin from a cancerous cyst of the kidney in a patient with renal carcinoma, helped confirm that the major source of the hormone in man was the kidney. Later, Wally Fried and Cliff showed that administration of androgens increased erythropoietin output and erythropoiesis—a finding that supported the administration of androgens to anemic patients with renal failure to diminish their transfusion requirement. Also, of great interest to me was Cliff's work related to the post-irradiation recovery of the stem cell pool as assessed by the response of the repopulated bone marrow to injections of partially purified erythropoietin.

Stem Cell Pool

Diana and I were working in the lab, when Cliff entered with a guest who had returned from a scientific meeting to Chicago with him. His guest looked to me like a Hungarian Hussar, spare, quick, chiseled facial features, thin rectangular spectacles—a heavy sport coat slung over one shoulder. I looked for a saber and a brace of pistols. He even had a Hungarian accent, apparent as Cliff introduced us to his friend, Dr. Laszlo Lajtha, from Oxford, England.

With little deference to casual conversation, Cliff and Laszlo mesmerized me with their theoretical concepts of the stem cell pool. They reasoned that the diminished numbers of radiosensitive stem cells repopulating sub-lethally irradiated bone marrow had to reproduce and replete the stem cell pool before they could respond to hormones, like erythropoietin, and differentiate into red blood cells. If these primitive progenitor cells did not reproduce to a given number first, there would not be enough to make white blood cells or platelets, to prevent sepsis or hemorrhage, needed to ensure survival.

Doris Gurney invited Karen and me to dine with Dr. Lajtha at the Gurney's that evening. Doris, a gracious hostess, lost no time interrogating Laszlo about his background in Hungary. He quickly corrected her, saying he had grown up in Transylvania, not Hungary.

His family lived in a mountainous region not far from a castle occupied by a count. Author Bram Stoker used him, Laszlo's neighbor, as his prototype for Count Dracula.

Laszlo told Doris about his grandfather's equipment for hunting bears—an iron bar and a long straight knife. His grandfather would confront a bear in the woods, hit him on the snout with the iron bar, and when the bear reared up on his two hind feet in pain and rage exposing his chest, grandfather lunged forth, thrusting home. Cliff said Laszlo's father was a symphony orchestra conductor in Paris. Laszlo had graduated from medical school in Budapest where one of his teachers was the 1937 Nobel Laureate in Medicine, Dr. Albert Szent-Gyorgyi, revered by his alumni.

Ten years later, inspired by Laszlo and Cliff's discussions of the elusive hemopoietic stem cell pool—with the help of Dr. William Osborne in his techniques of autoradiography, and with the expertise of Dr. John C. Hoak with his electron microscope—I was able to identify the hemopoietic stem cell in the irradiated mouse's bone marrow cell repopulated spleen colony.

Androgens

She wasn't wasted. She glowed with good health—not what we expected, seeing this attractive black woman in her forties with metastatic breast cancer. As a Hematology Fellow, I had brought my attending physician, Cliff Gurney, to see this patient in response to a request for consultation. She was not anemic, and surprisingly, her hematocrit was 56% (normal for female=42% +/- 5%). Her oncologist had prescribed testosterone injections to inhibit the action of female estrogens supporting the growth of the breast cancer cells, a recognized form of therapy in the 1960's. In another circumstance, hematologists had noted that some patients with aplastic anemia had responded to androgen therapy.

The normal male hematocrit levels of 47% +/- 5% are higher than the lower values in females, because, it was assumed, that estrogens tended to suppress erythropoiesis in females, and androgens enhanced erythropoiesis in males. I thought about this, wondering if by administering androgens to the six week-old Carworth Farms #1 female mice—used in the plethoric mouse bioassay system—would expand the stem cell pool and protect the bone marrow cells from the toxic of effect of radiation.

So I injected plethoric mice with testosterone enanthate for several days, and then I challenged them injecting a standard dose of six units of partially purified erythropoietin. The unexpected response was not from an enhanced uptake of red blood cell radio-iron 59 in the experimental group, but from the fact that the high hematocrit in the control group of mice injected with testosterone and saline, failed to suppress erythropoiesis as it usually did. I was conducting these experiments in Cliff's ACRH laboratory in 1963, and I could go no further, because I entered active duty in the U.S. Army Medical Corps at that time. After my service in the Army, I returned to ACRH to find that Wally Fried and Cliff—following up on my findings—had discovered the reason androgen injections induced erythropoiesis in mice. The injections of testosterone had increased the levels of erythropoietin in their blood.

Androgens and Renal Failure

This discovery came at an interesting time. Dr. Ray (Ardis) Lavender, one of my teachers, and my good friend, Dr. Marvin Forland, both faculty members in the Section of Nephrology, were caring for two patients with chronic renal failure. They required blood transfusions several times a month, because of the diseased kidneys in a Serbian minister, or lack of kidneys in the other patient, an aeronautical engineer, who had undergone total nephrectomy for hypertension. Both had low erythropoietin levels, too low to induce erythropoiesis to keep up with their anemia. I asked Gene Goldwasser, whose research group had partially purified erythropoietin, if they could provide the hormone for our proposed pilot study to reduce transfusions. They were unable to produce enough for our trial at the time. So, with informed consent by the patients, we undertook a pilot study to see if they would respond with a decreased transfusion requirement to a course of androgen therapy. In response to the androgens, the anephric engineer required fewer pints of blood, developed a good appetite, and gained body weight. The minister responded by no longer requiring transfused blood as his hematocrit rose, and he resumed an enthusiastic pursuit of his profession, preaching to the faithful in Chicago.

To complete our studies with androgens, and for the benefit of our patient study subjects, I deferred accepting my appointment as Associate Professor of Internal Medicine, Hematology and Radiation Research at The University of Iowa College of Medicine from the usual start time of 1 July until 1 December 1968. Six months later, Ray Lavender left The University of Chicago to become Director of Nephrology at Loyola College of Medicine and their Hines Veterans Hospital in western Chicago. Marv Forland left the U .of C. to accept a position as Director of Nephrology at The University of Texas, in San Antonio.

Studies with more patients by other investigators confirmed the benefits we observed, and nephrologists ministered androgens to their patients receiving renal dialysis for the next six years, until recombinant erythropoietin was released for therapy.

Algerians voted independence from France on 1 July 1962. President Charles de Gaulle, had presided over the French response to grant sovereignty to Algeria, and most French colonists, as many as 250,000, had departed Algeria by that time. This left a recalcitrant military group opposed to the separation, a terrorist organization, the Organization of Secret Army (OAS), raising havoc in a country now devoid of doctors who had left when the colonists departed. There were stories of OAS members rolling hand grenades down hospital corridors.

I was with Cliff Gurney, admiring the framed commendation by President John F. Kennedy hanging on his office wall, when I asked him to tell me about his experience in Algeria. With five other University of Chicago faculty members, Cliff had joined George V. Le Roy, MD, who had organized—under the aegis of Care Medico—a volunteer rescue mission to restore medical care to the people of Algiers.

When the volunteers from Chicago arrived in Algiers, Cliff said they could hear firing from the rebels in the hills around the city. You might ask what these professors, medical specialists, had to offer. Dr. Le Roy—a consummate organizer and diplomate—brought order out of chaos. Working with the local administrators and nurses, he got the hospital running again. Radiologist Nels Stranjord, MD, discovered a brand new Siemens X-Ray machine still in its shipping crate, because nobody knew how it worked. Nels unpacked it and got it operational. Before specializing in radiology and joining the Chicago faculty, Nels had been in the private general practice of medicine. He revived his skills, setting and casting fractured bones.

Cliff Gurney and his friend, John E. Kasik, MD, PhD, were hands-on doctors, but subspecialists in Internal Medicine—Cliff, a

Hematologist, John, a Pulmonologist, but they had the credentials for running the hospital's two pediatric wards. Cliff and Doris had five young children at home, and John and Sherle had six kids, who must have presented their doctor fathers with otitis media, sore throats, and all of the childhood xanthems. The Algerian children presented a problem requiring immediate attention. They were all crying at the top of their lungs. Within two days they stopped crying. I asked Cliff what treatments had John and he used to achieve silence. Cliff said, "We put screens on the windows to keep the biting insects out." After their month in Algiers, the Chicago contingent was replaced the following month by a similar group of volunteer doctors—faculty members from The University of Pennsylvania Medical School.

I met John Kasik in July 1960. He was my first attending physician when I started my residency in Internal Medicine at UCHC. We became friends, and ten years later, I helped recruit John to join us at The University of Iowa where he accepted a position as Professor of Internal Medicine in the Division of Pulmonary Medicine and Director of Oakdale, the state's Tuberculosis Sanitarium. His work on Isoniazid for his PhD in Pharmacology at Chicago put him out of one job, when he presided over the closing of Oakdale, but led to another, when he was appointed Chief of Staff of the Iowa City Veterans Administration Hospital, which was staffed by The University of Iowa faculty. He was also appointed Associate Dean of the College of Medicine.

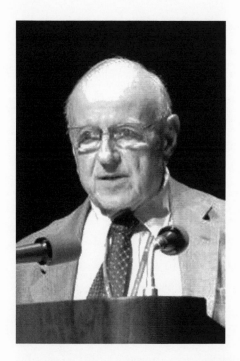

Sanford B. Krantz, MD

Mr. Elizaldi (fictional name) was admitted to the third floor of ACRH, a transfer from Costa Rica, arranged by our cardiologist, Dr. Fausto Tanzi, a native of San Jose', the capital of Costa Rica. Mr. Elizaldi, an accountant on a plantation in Costa Rica, of small stature, was bronzed from the many blood transfusions he had received to compensate for his lack of ability to make red blood cells. When the transfused red cells completed their life span, and were consumed by his macrophages, the iron from their hemoglobin was deposited in vital tissues. Excess iron in tissues injures organs like the pancreas and the heart. Our hematologists were asked to discover what caused the problem and solve it.

Pure Red Cell Aplasia

To help analyze the problem, Dr. Tanzi, who spoke fluent Spanish, was able to translate for us a history that revealed no particular exposure to toxins in the patient's job on the plantation. The examination of the sample of his bone marrow showed it was entirely bereft of erythroblasts, the precursors of red blood cells; an affliction called Pure Red Cell Aplasia. I performed a bioassay of the patient's plasma to find very elevated levels of erythropoietin in his blood, so the problem was that the bone marrow cells did not respond to the hormone and make red cells.

At the time, Sandy Krantz and I were new Assistant Professors of Internal Medicine in the Section of Hematology, our laboratories on the second floor of ACRH. Sandy, used a fluorescent antibody technique to demonstrate antibody adhering to a sample of the patient's primitive bone marrow cells. He concluded that Mr. Elizaldi had an autoimmune process suppressing his erythroblast precursors. In these days before the availability of specific immunosuppressive drugs, Sandy recommended that Mr. Elizaldi's attending physician prescribe a course of 6-mercaptopurine, an anti-leukemic drug known to be immunosuppressive. With the patient's informed consent, his attending physician prescribed a course of 6-MP, hoping to achieve a remission freeing him from dependence on blood transfusions to treat his anemia.

Blood counts were made every several days to see if the patient required a blood transfusion, and the technicians had never seen any reticulocytes in the blood smears. After about a week of therapy with 6-MP, the laboratory technician detected a shower of reticulocytes—new red blood cells—in Mr. Elizaldi's peripheral blood smear. This was followed by robust red blood cell production that obviated the need for transfusions. Moreover, the response to therapy was so vigorous that Mr. Elizaldi's physicians starting withdrawing pints of his blood to rid him of the excess iron he had accumulated over the months of transfusions.

Sandy was the first to discover Pure Red Cell Aplasia was an auto-immune disease, curable with immunosuprressive drugs. Results of that research, including his studies of erythropietin, meant such patients no longer required blood transfusions forever. He reported his work in over 200 scientific papers, and was elected to the American Society of Clinical Investigation and the Association of American Physicians.

In 1970, Sandy accepted a job as Chief of Hematology at Vanderbilt College of Medicine in Nashville, Tennessee, where he served for 24 years, building a strong division of hematology.

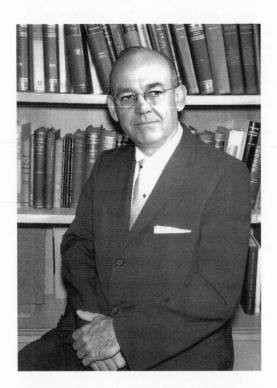

William E. Adams, MD

Dr. Adams deftly removed a rib with an Alexander periosteotome, permitting Don Kurlander and me to achieve wider exposure of the right chest with our retractors. Don was a pulmonary resident who had scrubbed in with us to assist in the surgery of his clinic patient. With the blood vessels and nerves left intact, the rib would grow back in the rib's sheath if the patient survived. As Dr. Adams proceeded with the pneumonectomy, he isolated and displayed a carcinoma the size of a lemon from the patient's right lung. Holding this large tumor in his gloved hand, he peered at Dr. Kurlander over the top of his spectacles above his surgical mask, to ask in a low serious voice, "Don, have you thought about giving up smoking cigarettes?"

Before 1930, attempts at removal of an entire lung for cancer—a pneumonectomy—had ended with the postoperative death of the patient. On leave from The University of Chicago in 1933, Dr. Adams served as principal assistant to Professor Evarts Graham, MD, of Washington University in St. Louis when Dr. Graham and he carried out the first successful pneumonectomy in a patient with lung cancer. Their patient lived for 18 years after the surgery to die of other causes.

As assistant professor of Surgery at The University of Chicago, Dr. Adams and his chief, Dr. Dallas B. Phemister, performed in 1938 the first one-step removal of the esophagus for cancer with restoration of the continuity of the digestive tract—technically, the first transthoracic esophagectomy and gastroesophagostomy in a patient with long survival. Subsequently, Dr. Adams developed other innovative techniques in thoracic surgery, later demonstrating patients can survive postoperatively with only 50% of lung tissue remaining after surgery, but he found that some patients with pulmonary hypertension were unable to withstand pneumonectomy.

Yosh Oda, my former medical school classmate, and I were assigned as interns to the Cardiovascular-Thoracic Surgical Service of Dr. Adams and Dr. Peter Moulder in September 1959. It was an exciting time at the beginning of open heart surgery. I gained insight into the problems surgeons faced when later I was consulted as a hematologist. My best memories are of Dr. Adams, a skillful master surgeon, a kind man with compassionate care of his patients.

Iowa to Chicago
William Elias Adams was born near Nichols, Iowa, on 1 May 1902 in rural Muscatine County. After graduating from West Liberty High School, he attended The University of Iowa. His mother died when he was ten years old, and his father died before he entered college.

After he graduated from The University of Iowa College of Medicine in 1926, he remained for two years as an instructor until his future bride Huberta M. Livingston (1905-1980) received her MD at Iowa in 1928. They married in her home in Hopkinton, Iowa on 9 June 1928. Following a surgical internship at Chicago's Presbyterian Hospital in 1932, Dr. (Livingston) Adams joined William Adams on the faculty, appointed Instructor in Surgery at The University of Chicago, and then Director of the Anesthesia Service in 1944, retiring in 1952.

Dr. William Adams advanced through the academic ranks in The University of Chicago School of Medicine with appointments as assistant professor of medicine in 1936, associate professor in 1940, professor in 1947, and finally, appointed to an endowed chair: James Nelson and Anna Louise Raymond Professor of Surgery. In 1967, he retired as Chairman of the Department of Surgery to serve for the next six years as assistant director of the American College of Surgeons with its headquarters in Chicago.

Dr. Adams's professional colleagues recognized his sense of duty and leadership over the years as they elected him President of the Chicago Medical Society and Vice President of the Illinois Medical Society. He was a founder of the American Board of Thoracic Surgery and President of the American Association of Thoracic Surgery and College of Chest Physicians. Appointed in 1965 as Chairman of the AMA Section of Diseases of the Chest, he also served as Secretary of the American College of Surgeons. He received many honors: Guest Assistant in Surgery at the University of Berlin (1935-1936), Honorary Professor of Surgery at the University of Guadalajara, recipient of Russia's Alexander B. Vishnevski's Medal. As a Fulbright Visiting Professor, he was invited to help develop cardiothoracic surgery at the Glasgow Royal Infirmary.

Not long after Karen Piper and I were married, we visited her mother and stepfather in their home in Decorah, Iowa. Karen pointed to a barely visible scar on her neck above her Adams apple and told me it was the site where Dr. William Adams had surgically removed a congenital thyroglossal duct cyst when she was four years old (1940). His wife, Dr. Huberta (Livingston) Adams had administered the anesthesia for the operation. Jan, Karen's mother, after listening to Karen's remarks, asked me, "How are Billy and Huberta?" I had no idea, and I think it was the first time I had heard of them. Jan went on to tell me that after Dr. William Adams graduated from medical school at Iowa in 1926, her first husband, Dr. Mark Piper, graduated in the next class in 1927, and Huberta Livingston graduated with her MD in 1928. The four became good friends while in school together in Iowa City.

Karen's mom must have called her friends, because after we returned to Chicago, Huberta Adams invited Karen and me to join them for supper at a local restaurant. Our first visit to the Adams's apartment in Hyde Park, near The University of Chicago campus was memorable, because we couldn't find it. We drove by the address we were given several times before we realized that the *Cloisters*, a gray four-story edifice with gothic arched doorways and a courtyard, was not a university building. A doorman in his red uniform with polished brass buttons quickly dissuaded us of that impression and welcomed us with, "You are expected." He escorted us on an elevator to the fourth floor. As the door opened Mrs. Adams greeted us with a broad smile, took our hands and ushered us into the foyer with parquet flooring leading to an immense beautiful high ceiling apartment. Her husband's welcoming warm smile supplemented hers to put us at ease. William Adams was slightly taller than Karen, maybe

5'9". His hair was thinning, but he had the square stocky frame of a vigorous man in his 50's. He looked fit.

After greetings and small talk, Mrs. Adams invited Karen and me to be their guests at a restaurant downtown. Dr. Adams donned a black cashmere coat, a gray homburg hat, and pearl gray gloves. He excused himself to retrieve his car from the garage. It was a shiny new black Cadillac, a gift from a grateful patient. Could his childhood friends from his hometown of Nichols, Iowa (population of 374), recognize their erstwhile playmate, now an internationally distinguished thoracic surgeon, perfectly at home in this thriving metropolis of more residents than in the State of Iowa?

Karen and I were the beneficiaries of the Adams's kindness and generosity. Shortly after our first meeting, during which we may have mentioned we were eating off a card table and using a steamer trunk and army blanket for a couch, in our unfurnished apartment #708, at 727 East 60th Street, we were summoned to the 14th floor of a wholesale furniture warehouse on Wabash Avenue. There, the owner, a grateful patient of Dr. Adams, directed us to pick out a lovely Duncan Phyfe-style dining room table and chairs, and a couch, which he sold and delivered to us at wholesale prices. When I was an intern on the Thoracic Surgery Service, Karen and I were invited with surgical house staff to the Adams's apartment for a reception and party, and for many times afterwards, they included us on their guest list for departmental parties.

HOPKINTON, IOWA

Huberta's childhood home in Hopkinton, Iowa, (population 681), was the Adams's escape from busy Chicago, their Shangri-La, where they found rest and recuperation. So in 1973, at Bill"s second retirement, the Adams returned after 45 years to live the rest of their lives in Iowa. Karen and I had been living in Iowa City where I was Professor of Internal Medicine at The University of Iowa. We looked forward to entertaining the Adams, hoping to return some of their hospitality as they planned to live only 70 miles from Iowa City. But Dr. Adams untimely death supervened.

I quote excerpts from a "Tribute to Dr. William E. Adams, prepared by Dr. Elam Davies, Pastor of the Fourth Presbyterian Church of Chicago (on Michigan Avenue across from Watertower Place) and presented by his assistant pastor at the funeral service in the First Presbyterian Church of Hopkinton, at 2:00 pm, Wednesday, 28 November 1973:

"...As I think of Dr. Adams, I think of a strong man who had a tender streak in his nature, a gentle man who would never hesitate to fight for the right and true. I recall him as a kindly person who expended himself far beyond the call of duty, who graciously led you to believe that what he did for you and others was the simplest act of concern, when you knew all along that it was costly compassion. He was self-effacing but never self-deprecating because he was confident in his expertise, and interlacing all these strands of his personality was a humility which had not the slightest trace of humbug about it."

Dr. Adams's pastor continued:

"He was one of those rare people who knew what he knew and knew what he didn't know,... To whatever task he gave himself he served selflessly and assiduously, never obtruding himself at the expense of others, but always there to be counted on, when others had, for one reason or another, left for the sidelines when the going was tough. He was always dignified but never pompous, always ready to praise without expecting a reciprocal backslap, always generous in his estimate of good being done without being falsely effusive..."

"...And I shall remember these things (his concern for others) when I think of him in connection with Fourth Church where as an elder for many years—'a tower of strength' to his pastor and friend to his fellow elders and members."

These words of Dr. Adams's pastor affected all of us who mourned the passing of this good man as we sat in the pews of Hopkinton's First Presbyterian Church and thought about our past associations on that cold, overcast November day.

Friends and Colleagues

In addition to the many of the Adams's friends from Hopkinton, friends and colleagues from around the country came to fill the church and pay their respect. Dr. Peter V. Moulder from Gainesville, Florida was joined by the other casket bearers, all cardiothoracic surgeons from Colorado, Michigan, Tennessee, Pennsylvania, and Illinois. My former intern partner, Dr. Willard Fry, a cardiac surgeon from Chicago, greeted me after a separation of 12 years. Of the honorary casket bearers, Obstetrician Dr. Charles P. McCartney, President of the Chicago Medical Society, had delivered my first son, Robert, 11 years previously in Chicago Lying-In Hospital. Other honorary casket bearers included Dr. Adams's former residents, physicians representing the American College of Surgeons (its director), the Illinois State Medical Society, The University of Chicago Faculty, and the American Association of Thoracic and Cardiovascular Surgeons.

After the service, Karen and I walked under a gray November sky threatening snow to the Adams home for the reception. Huberta, with daughter Diana at her side, brightened the day with her warm smile I recalled from our first meeting 18 years ago. We stepped over the threshold of her immaculate old Victorian house to warmth and reflection. Huberta had grown up in this house, the home of Hopkinton's Doctor Livingston and his family. When few women went to college, and fewer attended medical school, Huberta excelled at her education and later as an academic anesthesiologist at The University of Chicago. Dr. William Barclay, former Chief of the Pulmonary Section at Chicago, and later, Editor of the Journal of the American Medical Association, wrote in his memorial tribute that Huberta had researched anesthetic drugs, designed anesthetic equipment, and published more than 150 scientific papers. She had been elected President of the Chicago Society of Anesthesiologists, the Illinois Society of Anesthesiologists, and the Midwestern Association of Anesthesiologists. She was a remarkably talented woman who bore her grief with courage.

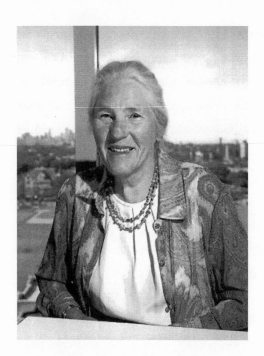

Janet D. Rowley, MD

One day in 1965, a tall attractive woman with dark hair, wearing a white coat, moved—with the help of her technician—a microscope and sterile hood, into an empty laboratory at the far end of the second floor of ACRH. Cliff Gurney introduced her to me as Dr. Janet Rowley, who joined us in the Section of Hematology. Cliff said she had returned from a year in England, working with his friend, Dr. Laszlo Lajtha, learning how to karyotype the chromosomes of bone marrow cells. She would be analyzing portions of bone marrow specimens our patients permitted us to use for research studies of diseases of the blood and bone marrow.

Janet and her technician grew bone marrow cells in tissue culture, arresting them in mitosis, isolating their 48 chromosomes, arranging them according to standard classification, and preparing a photomicrograph of them; a karyotype. Janet discovered a consistent 22-9 translocation of the Philadelphia chromosome in bone marrow cells of our patients with chronic myelocytic leukemia, which she believed caused the disease. Later, she discovered a consistent 21-8 translocation in the bone marrow cells of patients with acute myeloblastic leukemia. Her findings, and those of others, confirmed that cancer was a genetic disease.

Other investigators discovered that the activity of the BCR-ABL fusion protein—that caused the translocation of 22-9 of the Philadelphia chromosome—could be blocked by a tyrosine kinase inhibitor, imatinib (Gleevec) to induce a remission in patients with chronic myelocytic leukemia. Prescription of Gleevec to patients with chronic myelocytic leukemia—afflicting patients 25 to 60 years of age—extended their remissions from a median survival of 2 ½ years, to decades. If patients taking Gleevec underwent remission for 2 years, they experienced the same life expectancy as persons without cancer.

Janet graduated from The University of Chicago School of Medicine in 1949, long before women made up 50% of medical school classes in the United States. In addition to publishing 500 scientific papers, she and her husband, Donald A. Rowley, MD, Professor of Pathology, raised three sons. Janet and Don graciously hosted a reception in their home in Hyde Park for members of the Section of Hematology including Karen and me. It was an opportunity to get to know the Rowley's in a casual setting where Karen and I found them warm and welcoming.

Janet's work was recognized with her promotion to an endowed professorship, receipt of the Lasker award, and the Presidential Medal of Fredom—presented by President Barack Obama. Yale and Harvard awarded her honorary degrees. She was elected to the National Academy of Sciences, among other prestigious honors.

The last time I saw Janet, and had an opportunity to speak with her, was at the symposium in honor of Dr. Jacobson in 1992. During her talk, she modestly thanked Jake for giving her—an untried investigator—an opportunity to pursue work in a new field by making her appointment to the ACRH. Later, I read in the alumni bulletin that she continued to attend her laboratory well into her 80's, pedaling her bicycle to the hospital from her home in Hyde Park. She died at age 88 on 17 December 2013.

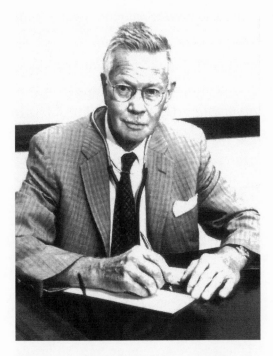

Henry T. Ricketts, MD

As I entered an examining room in the Diabetes-Metabolism Clinic with Dr. Ricketts, his patient greeted him like an old friend. Dr. Ricketts introduced me as his resident, and asked the patient how he had been getting along. Thereafter, I watched him, a master clinician, review the patient's diet and general history, and perform a thorough physical examination. In addition to examining his fundi with an ophthalmoscope, listening to his heart and lungs, and palpating his abdomen, he spent time examining the patient's feet and toes for signs of vascular insufficiency, neuropathy, and gangrene. A consummate teacher, his patient and I benefitted from his efforts.

Tight Control

In the days before technology permitted patients with diabetes and their doctors to obtain instant results of the blood sugar and A-1C tests, blood samples were analyzed at the clinic visit, and 24-hour urine specimens collected at home, were tested for sugar to regulate the schedule for insulin administration. In the 1960's, diabetologists separated into two camps: tight control of blood sugars, versus laissez-faire—let the patient do what he felt like doing. Dr. Ricketts kept detailed records of test results, and practiced tight control of blood and urine sugars, later proven to prevent or delay the onset of blindness, vascular insufficiency, and chronic renal failure.

With excellent nurses, Dr. Ricketts efficiently ran the Diabetes-Metabolism Service with his junior partner, Dr. Henry L. Wildberger, a 1951 graduate of The University of Chicago. Dr. Ricketts was reserved, spare, quick, and of slightly less than average height, in contrast to his partner, Dr. Wildberger, who was a large man—over six feet tall—talkative, with an easy laugh, who sometimes ignored his page over the hospital's public address system. So, the fun-loving women operators repeated again and again, "Calling Doctor Henry *Worthington* Wildberger," using a middle name they made up to get his attention.

When he was only nine years old, Henry Ricketts lost his father— one of medicine's heroes. His father, Howard Taylor Ricketts (1871-1910), a pathologist on the faculty of The University of Chicago, died in Mexico City of typhus, a disease he was studying. Typhus was caused by one of the organisms named for him, a rickettsia. Familiar to most physicians is the organism that causes Rocky Mountain spotted fever—*Rickettsia rickettsii*. Henry Ricketts graduated from Harvard Medical School. He was one of the original clinical faculty members of The University of Chicago shortly after clinical services arrived on the South Side of Chicago at the university's new Albert Merritt Billings Hospital (AMBH).

I do not know who assigned each of us as freshmen classmates, to a faculty advisor during our first days of orientation. We were given appointments to meet our advisor and establish a relationship to last four years until graduation. One of my friends met with his advisor, a professor of Internal Medicine, before I met mine. My classmate said the meeting was cordial during which his advisor said, "Come and see me if you have a problem." In four years, my friend never experienced a problem that rose to that level.

MY ADVISOR

The memo I received listed Dr. Henry Ricketts, as my advisor with the time of my appointment and his office number where I could meet him. When I arrived at his office, his secretary said, "Dr. Ricketts is working in the lab down the hall. He is expecting you, and he wants you to meet him there." I found the lab and Dr. Ricketts, who had just finished operating on an anesthetized experimental animal. He was in his undershorts changing out of scrubs to put on his trousers. Thinking nothing of his informal attire, he greeted me and said he liked to invite the students assigned to him, one from each class, to join him for dinner later in the fall.

Around 5:00 pm on a nice fall day in November, I donned sport coat, slacks, and tie, and left my room in Burton-Judson Court, (the graduate student dormitory) anticipating a pleasant evening and dinner at the Ricketts's home. I found their four-story brick row house on Kenwood, a lovely tree-lined street north and east of The University of Chicago campus. Dr. Ricketts answered the doorbell with a perplexed look on his face. To my great embarrassment, I learned my mistake. The dinner was *next* week.

The next week, when Dr. Ricketts opened the front door of his home, he saw me, a bedraggled, sorry-looking soul, with a sheepish look on my face, having walked from the dormitory in the rain. He led me into the foyer, hung up my dripping rain coat, sat me in front of the fireplace with a warm fire, bade me take off my shoes, and handed me an Old Fashion cocktail.

Soon, we were joined by the three other medical students, (a sophomore, junior, and senior) assigned to Dr. Ricketts. After introductions and libations, we were treated to a special dinner that Mrs. Ricketts and their maid prepared and served. Earlier that week, Dr. Ricketts had hunted wild duck on the Mississippi River, and we were the beneficiaries of his skills in the duck blind. Each year thereafter, I looked forward to this special dinner, enjoying the Ricketts's gracious hospitality and meeting the new freshman medical student assigned to our host. This year, it was Randolph Seed. Randy was the son of Chicago surgeon, Dr. Lindon Seed. The director of the blood bank, Dr. Lindon Seed, had in 1937 invited my father to see the nation's first blood bank, established in 1936 by Bernard Fantus in the Cook County Hospital.

During the summer, Dr. Ricketts had taken up barbecuing over a charcoal grill in his small enclosed back yard. The beef tasted so good, cooked over the fire, he decided to grill steaks inside during the winter months. So he brought the grill into the basement and jerry-rigged a fan and duct system to exhaust the heat. He wished to treat us, his student guests, to his especially barbecued steaks. After an hour of libations and conversation, he donned an apron and descended to the basement to cook for us. All seemed to go well for about twenty minutes. Then we heard footsteps racing up the basement stairs. The kitchen the door flew open and Dr. and Mrs. Ricketts, and the maid emerged, coughing, in a cloud of smoke. Fortunately, the conflagration was well confined. The windows were opened to air out the kitchen and dining room, and the party proceeded in good humor.

The Ricketts's annual dinner in November 1960 was memorable. After a delicious meal, Karen and I, and a couple of other medical students and their wives gathered around the piano in the living room. Mrs. (Mandy) Ricketts played the piano, Dr. Ricketts played a sailor's concertina, and we joined them to sing sea chanteys. The Ricketts had returned that fall from competing in the Mackinac Races, sailing their sloop *Norther* in Lake Michigan from Chicago to Mackinac Island and back. We learned they would dry the *Norther's* sails, hanging them in the four-story-high stairwell opposite the front door. They loved sailing the inland waters.

Asked to wait until our fellow students had departed, the Ricketts told us their plans for a vacation in the spring. They had chartered a sailboat and crew for a month to sail the Aegean and Mediterranean Seas, visiting the Greek Islands. Would we stay in their home while they were gone, they asked?

Abandoning our one bedroom apartment to live in the luxurious space of the Ricketts's townhouse, and eat suppers prepared by their maid, was an offer we couldn't refuse. We were not just house-sitting. I am sure Henry and Mandy asked us to be there, because Nancy, their teenage daughter, would be staying at home attending her senior year in high school. Until we met Nancy, we wondered if we were there to chaperone wild parties of irresponsible adolescents. We need not have been concerned, because Nancy was mature beyond her years, studying, practicing on the piano—a well-organized, highly intelligent, nice person, like her mother.

The Ricketts's son, Dr. Howard Ricketts, and his wife, joined us and others for dinner to welcome the sailors, tanned and a little tired, home from their month sailing vacation. In conversation, I happened to mention that the Senior Scientific Session was scheduled for that evening. Henry said he had forgotten the date, and despite just having returned from a trip of several thousand miles, left with me after dinner to attend, duty-bound, the Session in P-117. He joined a number of other members of the faculty that night to support the senior medical students by discussing their presentations of the research they had undertaken during the year.

Henry was brisk, not brusque, in his speech as he talked to patients and medical students, but when Karen and I were in his home on Kenwood, he relaxed, and his conversation relaxed. Before Christmas one year, the Ricketts accepted our invitation for dinner in our small apartment. Mrs. Ricketts was admiring the Christmas cards Karen had displayed on our windowsill, when she accidentally knocked them on the floor. Without hesitation, this beautiful, dignified woman laughingly apologized and was on her hands and knees retrieving the cards, despite our protests. We exchanged Christmas cards with the Ricketts for several years after Karen and I left Chicago for Iowa City. One of their cards contained a photo of Henry and Mandy, then is their 60's, smiling, on skis, in the Rocky Mountains. We were not surprised.

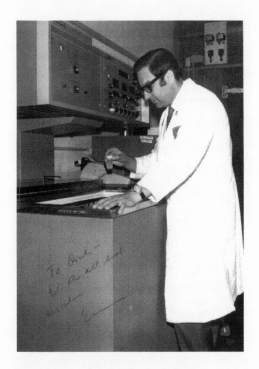

Ernest Beutler, MD

I regret that I never asked Ernie why he decided to measure gluta-thione in primaquine-sensitive red cells, leading him to discover—therein—diminished levels of reduced glutathione (GSH).

Radiobiology flourished in the 1950's as scientists learned about how ionizing radiation induced the formation of oxygen-dependent intracellular short-lived free radicals that sliced through DNA, pre-venting cells from replicating and repairing themselves, killing them. Concerned about fallout of radioactive isotopes from atomic bombs blasts, the scientists sought to protect cells from damage by free rad-icals, and found that compounds containing sulfhydryl groups (like GSH), served as free radical scavengers, anti-oxidants. They thought that if a potential victim of an atomic blast could swallow a pill con-taining sulfhydryl groups, he might survive death from radiation.

Lieutenant Ernest Beutler, U.S. Army Medical Corps, a 1950 Chicago medical school graduate—assigned in 1953 to The University of Chicago-Army Medical Research Project—worked with University of Chicago biochemist, Dr. Guzman-Barone, an expert on sulfhydryl metabolism, to study how red blood cells were protected from free radicals arising from the action of oxidant drugs, like primaquine. Ernie's discovery of decreased levels of GSH in the red cells of persons who sustained a hemolytic episode after ingesting the antimalarial drug, primaquine, led to the later discovery—by Dr. Paul E.Carson, his successor on the Project—of Glucose-6-Phosphate Dehydrogenase (G-6-PD) Deficiency. If a physician knew of this inherited enzyme defect, using tests developed on the Project, he could warn his patient to avoid primaquine and other oxidant drugs that might produce a hemolytic anemia.

Ernie's lectures on clinical diagnosis to my sophomore class were the epitome of clarity and logic. He lectured without notes, yet his lectures could have been published verbatim without a need for editing. I fondly remember his response to a colleague who challenged his declaration about the invariable characteristic of a blood disease by saying, "We see this sometimes."

In 1959, Ernie accepted the job as Chairman of Internal Medicine at the City of Hope National Medical Center in Duarte, California. Children with galactosemia are unable to metabolize the galactose sugar in milk. Ernie developed a test to detect the defect in newborns. He purified the enzyme in another inherited defect, Tay-Sachs disease. An associate, Dr. Karl Blume, and he published the first paper using a bone marrow transplant from a volunteer relative to treat a patient with leukemia.

Ernie moved to Scripps Research Institute in La Jolla, California in 1978. There, he isolated the gene for Gaucher's Disease, a lipid-storage disease, developed a test for the disease and improved its treatment. He developed cladribine, a drug to treat leukemia and multiple sclerosis.

In his spare time from being a father of a daughter and three sons, doing research, writing 800 scientific papers, book chapters and monographs, he developed the software, Reference Manager. One of Ernie's sons, Dr. Bruce Beutler, was his colleague at Scripps. He received the 2011 Nobel Prize in Medicine. Ernie died in 2008 of malignant lymphoma before he could proudly celebrate his son's award.

Affirmative Action

When I served on the Admissions Committee of The University of Iowa College of Medicine, committee members were charged with admitting 20% of the incoming class from an "underserved" population, Blacks and Hispanics. I remember Ernie telling me his concern about affirmative action—using quotas to select students for admission to medical school—because in the 1920's, quotas were used to ensure that no more than 20% of Jewish students would make up a medical school class. I was fond of my 72 classmates, and I got to know most of them pretty well, because of our small class. While I was in school, it never occurred to me to wonder about it, but after I thought about Ernie's remarks years after graduating, I looked at my class picture, remembering conversations with my friends, to note about half my class members were Jewish.

Ernest Beutler was born in Berlin on 30 September 1928. In 1935, at age seven, he immigrated to Milwaukee with his family—his mother and father were Jewish physicians—to escape persecution in Hitler Germany. After two years of high school, he entered The University of Chicago in a special program, where he received his bachelor's degree in 1948. Two years later, in 1950, he received his MD from that esteemed institution.

As an intern on the Hematology Service, I worked with Dr. Beutler shortly before he left for California. I was taking care of Zena Books (fictional name), a 22-year old black woman. She had been admitted to our service on the third floor of ACRH for a painful crisis and to heal an ulcer on her ankle, both a result of her sickle cell disease. She was admitted to the hospital every six to eight weeks for therapy with analgesics, intravenous fluids, and blood transfusions to treat the effects of her inherited sickle cell (SS) hemoglobin. When a critical number of red blood cells with SS hemoglobin are deprived of oxygen, they clump, obstruct blood flow in fine blood vessels, cause severe pain, and death of tissues.

Red blood cells containing methemoglobin do not bind oxygen, and Ernie thought they might buffer cells with sickle hemoglobin to prevent them from clumping. Dr. Beutler reasoned that if he could make 20% of Zena's red cells contain methemoglobin, it might interrupt the process that caused her so much distress and so many hospitalizations. So, with Zena's consent, she received increasing doses of sodium nitrate to produce methemoglobinemia. We were not able to achieve an optimal level of methemoglobin, and we terminated the study. I recall this anecdote to show how Ernie, using his knowledge of pathophysiology, strived to relieve his patient's pain and suffering.

After Dr. Beutler became head of research at Scripps, he produced a week-long course in Hematology-Oncology, every February at Torrey Pines in La Jolla, California. He had no difficulty attracting the top experts from the snowy states in the east to lecture to an eager audience. Attending this excellent program provided an opportunity for me to review and sharpen clinical skills, and a chance to speak with my friend and medical hero.

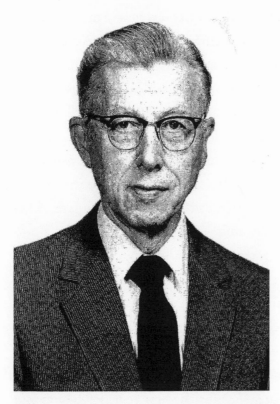

Kenneth M. Brinkhous, MD

I reached for the ringing telephone. The bedside clock glowed 2:00 am. After listening to my Hematology Fellow on the other end of the line, I said, "Order the tests, stat." Now awake, Karen asked, "What?" "We have a hematology consultation. Sorry to wake you, I'll see you later," I responded. Within the hour, I found my way to the Surgical Intensive Care Unit at The University of Iowa Hospitals and Clinics, a trip I could make in my sleep, I had been there so many times. But now I was wide awake.

It was fortunate our patient was intubated and asleep, because watching the nurse removing the blood-soaked dressings from his surgical incision might lead him to conclude he could bleed to death. Blood was dripping rapidly in his intravenous tubing from the tenth unit of blood from the blood bank. My fellow and I were there partly because of the implied, but unstated suggestion to the patient's doctor by Dr. Ronald Strauss (Director of the Elmer L. DeGowin Blood Center), "If you want any more blood for your patient, request a Hematology Consultant to stop the bleeding.

By now the results from the tests I had asked my fellow to order were back. So we were able to ascertain which components of the hemostatic (blood clotting) mechanism were deficient and needed to be replaced. My hematology colleagues and I had developed a protocol for measuring, in a prescribed schedule, the effects of infusing the missing blood components to clot the blood and stop the massive hemorrhage. Implementing the protocol worked, and the patient did not die of "complications of surgery."

We were able to help this patient survive because of the discoveries of Dr. Kenneth Brinkhous, his colleagues and of those of other investigators. Contemplate, if you will, how remarkably complex the body's system of blood clotting evolved to stop bleeding from wounds or menses, yet then stopped the clotting to prevent thrombosis (clots) in blood vessels that would lead to hypoxia of tissues and gangrene. Dr. Robert MacFarlane, Regius Professor of Medicine at the Radcliffe Infirmary of The University of Oxford, England—father of my friend and colleague, Dr. Donald MacFarlane—brought order to our thinking about the dozen factors in plasma that acted to form a blood clot after a wound. He stated the progressive proteolysis of these proteins acted as a cascade from a wound, releasing tissue factor, to the subsequent activation of each factor in sequence to convert fibrinogen to fibrin, making a clot.

Kenneth Brinkhous was born in Clayton County Iowa on 29 May 1908. He graduated from Central High School in Elkader, Iowa, in 1925, and he is listed in their Hall of Fame. Platted in 1846, Elkader, this town of 1200 citizens, nestled in the valley of the Turkey River in Northeast Iowa, is named for Emir Abd el-Kader, a young Algerian hero, a resistance fighter against French colonialism from 1836-1847. Who would have guessed?

IOWA

Ken secured an appointment to West Point, but he left the U.S. Military Academy, to matriculate at The University of Iowa in Iowa City, because he wanted to study medicine. He graduated with his BA in 1929 and with his MD from The University of Iowa College of Medicine in 1932.

At Iowa, he joined a group of pathologists engaged in research on blood coagulation, including Drs. Emory Warner, Homer Smith, Seegers and Owen, who discovered Vitamin K and its role in blood clotting. Dr. Brinkhous discovered that patients with hemophilia failed to make a component of the blood clotting system—he called it anti-hemophilic factor (AHF), later named Factor VIII—necessary for blood to coagulate.

He entered World War II as a medical officer, serving on the staff of General Douglas MacArthur in Australia, where he set up a reference laboratory for the Pacific Theater of Operations. Discharged from the Army as a Lieutenant Colonel, he returned to his family and their home at 1210 Yewell Street in Iowa City. He rented the house from Howard Moffitt, like my home at 1218 Yewell Street—three bedrooms, one bathroom, attached garage, furnished, at $32.50 per month. My father frequently remarked about what a fine investigator our neighbor was, whom I first met before the war, when I was probably six years old. I was eleven when he returned from service. I remember this kind man took time to talk to the kids in the neighborhood, and we were sorry to see him leave for North Carolina.

In the 1970's, our young male patients with hemophilia, admitted to our hematology service at The University of Iowa Hospitals and Clinics, rarely survived beyond their 20's, because of the morbidity caused by their bleeding diathesis. Initially, we infused fresh frozen plasma that contained AHF to stop bleeding episodes. Then Dr. Judith Poole, an Iowa graduate on the faculty at Stanford, discovered that the precipitate left in the near empty bag of fresh frozen plasma at the end of the infusion, contained a highly concentrated source of Factor VIII. Using cryoprecipitate—as it was called—permitted us to greatly reduce the volume of fluid infused to achieve hemostasis, avoiding heart failure from volume overload of the cardiovascular system. Cryoprecipitate (cryo=cold) could be prepared and stored in blood banks for patients with hemophilia. Of course, treatment with pure Factor VIII would provide optimal therapy. As a result of these discoveries, by the 1980's the 10,000 male persons in the United States could expect to live a normal life span.

NORTH CAROLINA

In 1946, Dr. Brinkhous accepted an invitation to become Chief of Pathology and Laboratory Medicine at The University of North Carolina, in Chapel Hill. There he worked tirelessly to untangle the complex process that causes blood to clot. He purified Factor VIII to improve therapy of hemophilia, and to study the genetic predisposition to that disease and other hemorrhagic diatheses, like Factor IX deficiency (Christmas Disease), and Von Willebrand Disease. He wrote 450 papers for peer-reviewed scientific, journals, books, and reports.

Hemophilia plagued the male members of Queen Victoria's royal family, passed from unaffected female carriers of the gene to males. In order to understand inheritance of the disease and to help develop gene therapy, Dr. Brinkhous studied a colony of dogs, deficient in Factor VIII, another group deficient in Factor IX, and a colony of pigs with Von Willebrand Disease.

In addition to his research, Ken mentored many young doctors, designed laboratory facilities for new hospitals, and served his profession as President of the American Medical Association (1955-56), the American Society for Experimental Pathology (1965-66), and the Federation of American Societies for Experimental Biology (1966-67).

HONORS AND AWARDS

For his work, Dr. Brinkhous received honorary doctoral degrees from The University of North Carolina and The University of Chicago. He was elected to the American Academy of Arts and Sciences and to the National Academy of Sciences. He served as President of the American Society of Investigative Pathologists and received its Gold-Headed Cane Award in 1981. The National Institutes of Health recognized him as the recipient of the longest (50 years) continuous extramural grant award (1947-1997).

Before I attended the scientific sessions at the annual December meeting of the American Society of Hematology, and before Karen, my wife, went Christmas shopping, we had breakfast in the headquarters hotel coffee shop. I introduced Karen to Ken Brinkhous, who had come there alone for breakfast. Karen was a native of Northeast Iowa, like Ken. He asked about my parents, the crops in Northeast Iowa and about what happened to the 12 or so doctors—his former neighbors who lived in Howard Moffitt's affordable housing on Yewell Street. He was a warm, friendly person, loved by his colleagues and students at North Carolina. He served as Chief of the Department of Pathology and Laboratory Medicine from 1946 to 1973, and attended his research laboratory until the year before he died at the age of 92, on 11 December 2000.

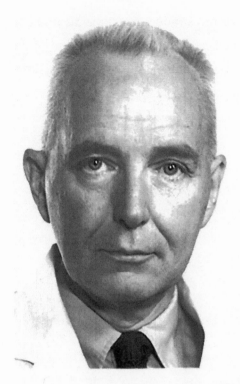

Charles B. Huggins, MD

Observers who did not know him may have felt it was undignified for Dr. Charles Huggins, a professor holding an endowed chair in medicine, to display a plaque above his laboratory door, ***Discovery is Our Business***. However, it was hard to belittle the discoveries this plain-speaking man made that led to the relief of pain and suffering of men and women afflicted with cancer. We were thrilled to learn his brilliance and hard work for the past 30 years would be recognized when it was announced he would share the 1966 Nobel Prize in Medicine with Dr. Peyton Rous of the Rockefeller Institute. In an interview with a *Chicago Tribune* reporter, he praised his wife's support through his life of research, proclaiming no bachelor could win the Prize.

Perhaps many persons knew of the work by his co-recipient of the prize, Dr. Peyton Rous, who had demonstrated that cancer could be caused by a virus, as in his namesake, Rous Sarcoma Virus. But I wonder how many knew of the connection he had with another member of the medical faculty at The University of Chicago, Oswald H. Robertson, MD.

Before World War I, Peyton Rous mentored Oswald H. Robertson, MD, working in his laboratory at the Rockefeller Institute, to develop a solution to preserve whole blood for transfusion. When World War I broke out in Europe, Dr. Robertson joined the British Army Medical Corps and set up the first blood bank in history, publishing the results of his work in the British Medical Journal in 1919, after the war.

Sometime in the 1940's my father presented results of his research on the preservation and transport of whole blood at a scientific meeting in Chicago in which he gave credit to the earlier work of Robertson and Rous. He thought Robertson long dead, but Dr. Robertson arose from the audience and discussed my father's paper. In the definitive work, *Blood Transfusion*, by Drs. Elmer L. DeGowin, Robert C. Hardin and John B. Alsever, my dad dedicated the book as follows:

"To Peyton Rous and Joseph R. Turner
Whose Basic studies at the Rockefeller Institute in
1915 made the Preservation of Blood a Reality
and to
Oswald H. Robertson
Who, in British Casualty Clearing Stations in France
in 1917, Conceived and Operated the First Blood Bank
This Book is Respectively Dedicated"

ORCHIECTOMY

I think Cliff Gurney first told me the story of Dr. Huggins's discovery. Dr. Huggins was one of the eight early members of the full-time faculty of The University of Chicago on the South Side campus, where he had the time to undertake laboratory research on the physiology of the urologic system without the stringent demands of a busy clinical practice. In the course of his studies, he catheterized the seminal vesicles of dogs and analyzed the seminal fluid to find it contained high levels of acid phosphatase. After he performed an orchiectomy (castration), he discovered that the elevated levels of acid phosphatase in the dogs' seminal fluid had markedly decreased.

He knew that patients with metastatic prostate cancer had high levels of acid phosphatase in their blood. When a patient, bedridden with pain from advanced prostate cancer, metastatic to bone, sought care at the University of Chicago Hospitals and Clinics, Dr. Huggins and his urology resident, Dr. Cornelius Vermeulen, examined the patient and told him he might benefit from orchiectomy, based on the research they had performed. The patient requested they proceed with the operation, and his doctors performed the first orchiectomy on a patient with advanced prostate cancer. In a few days, the patient got out of bed saying his pain had greatly diminished. His doctors credited the operation with remarkable psychological effects. As the patient continued to improve over the next several months, x-rays of his bones showed the metastases had shrunk. He died twelve years later of a stroke. Four of the 21 patients with prostate cancer Dr. Huggins treated with anti-androgen therapy lived for 12 years after treatment.

Coinvestigator Elwood Jensen, PhD, working with Dr. Huggins, studied female laboratory rats that developed breast cancers when given, an aromatic polycylic hydrocarbon (dimethylbenzanthrasate (DMBA or "Deembah!" as Dr. Huggins called it). Dr. Jensen discovered estrogen receptors on breast tissue and uterine tissue. When the receptors were blocked with anti-estrogen agents, the cancers underwent atrophy. His work provided additional support for the idea that cancers arising from endocrine tissue were dependent on hormone stimulation for their growth, and blocking the hormone receptors introduced the development of new therapy for such tumors. As a result, breast cancer can be classified as estrogen receptor positive or negative to guide therapy.

Charles Bretton Huggins was born in Canada on 22 September 1901, five days before my father was born across the border in Michigan. After he earned a BA degree from Acadia University, Dr. Huggins attended Harvard Medical School where he graduated at age 22. From 1924 until 1927, he served an internship and residency in general surgery at the University of Michigan with the renowned surgeon Dr. Frederick A. Coller.

My father, who received his MD from Michigan in 1928, recalled seeing Dr. Huggins enter a classroom and walk half-way up the aisle toward the lecturer. The lecturer paused to see what he wanted. My father and his medical classmates looked up from taking notes when Dr. Huggins remembered whatever he was thinking, turned around, and walked out. My dad told me this story when I mentioned I was listening to a distinguished visiting speaker in the conference room of ACRH, when Dr. Huggins suddenly stood up from his seat in the third row of the audience, and without saying a word, walked out.

I recall meeting Dr. Huggins three times. The first: I was a senior medical student, assigned to the Urology Out-clinic, in the course of presenting a patient's interim history and physical findings in a conference room to his physician, Dr. Cornelius Vermeulen, Chief of Urology, when Dr. Huggins interrupted me to ask, "What is alkaline phosphatase?" After the first three words of my answer, he said, "You sound like a lawyer," and walked out of the room.

The second: Cliff Gurney dispatched me as his resident to ask Dr. Huggins if he could offer a new medication for one of our patients with advanced cancer for whom we had run out of therapeutic options. I waited until Dr. Huggins finished berating a urology resident for taking more than twenty minutes to perform a skin-to-skin nephrectomy. He took the x-rays of the patient I had brought with me, slapped them up on the view box, looked at them for less than a minute and said, "Nothing can be done." I started to ask a question, but the flip of his fingers told me, "Be gone." I was dismissed.

Third: I was summoned to Dr. Huggins's office, not knowing what to expect, where I found him talking to my Uncle Ralph. Dr. Huggins greeted me like a long lost son, all smiles, with compliments about what a good resident I was. Ralph was there as the assistant to Dr. Endicott, in charge of extramural grants of the National Cancer Institute, to schedule a site visit for advisors to review a grant application Dr. Huggins had submitted to the NCI.

In addition to the Nobel Prize, Dr. Huggins won more than 100 awards, including the Cameron Prize for Therapeutics of the University of Edinburgh, and election to the National Academy of Sciences. Justly proud of the recognition of his work, Cliff Gurney told me Dr. Huggins referred to Urology as "Queen of the Medical Sciences." Dr. Huggins died in on 12 January 1997 at the age of 95.

A STORY OF HOPE

Dr. Huggins and Dr. Jensen discovered that cancers arising from certain tissues required hormonal stimulation to thrive. In the case of prostate cancer, when androgen stimulation was curtailed, or when testosterone receptors on prostate tissue were blocked by therapeutic agents, the cancer would cease to grow and even atrophy. I told this story of Dr. Huggins's discoveries to my oncologist, at The University of Iowa Cancer Center, Rohan Garje, M.D. when I thanked him for applying treatment based on Dr. Huggins's work to my care, permitting me to enjoy a remission long enough to finish writing this piece.

Acknowledgements

My son Bill keeps me focused on my work and my life, communicating frequently by telephone, e-mail and by overnight visits. I have no words good enough to thank him for his kindness.

I give special thanks to my friends who have read a draft of the typescript and have suggested changes improving the narrative. Bill O'Connor, a Chicagoan and Northeast Iowan, brought his special perspective and nuanced observations of the work to my attention. Thanks, Bill. Margaret Nelson has embellished with her red pen nearly every page of the typescript lending clarity and grace to the work with the skill and knowledge of a seasoned editor. Thanks, Margie.

My colleagues, Robin, Ben, and Shirley, and I benefited from the founders of the Malaria Project, our predecessors, Lowell T. Coggeshall, MD, and Alf Sven Alving, MD. It provided an opportunity for our inmate volunteers and for us to find redemption, payback, in service to our country and to persons living in tropics where multi-drug resistant malaria was endemic.

From 1963 until 1965, a time that will never be repeated, our work was supported by the enlightened leadership of the Surgeon General of the U.S. Army, General Robert C. Blount, MC, the Dean of The University of Chicago School of Medicine, Leon O. Jacobson, MD, and the Warden of Stateville Penitentiary, Frank J. Pate.

By 1970, the Malaria Project had been discontinued, at the beginning of an era of "get tough on crime" and "stop coddling criminals," in which inmates could not be required to work in prison industries or permitted to benefit from vocational training and educational programs, as before.

Reading history informs us that attitudes and trends cycle over time, so with the current interest in prison reform, we can hope that rehabilitation will once again receive emphasis over punishment.

FOR BOOK TWO:

My thanks to Charles E. Platz, MD ('63MD), Professor Emeritus of Pathology, Chief of Surgical Pathology, University of Iowa College of Medicine. He read the typescript of this work and made suggestions for its improvement. As a graduate of The University of Chicago, he knew the doctors of the stories, helping to correct my imperfect memory.

I am grateful to Robert E. Rakel, MD, Professor Emeritus, Founding Chairman, Department of Family Medicine, at Iowa and later at the Baylor School of Medicine, Houston, Texas, for reviewing the typescript, and suggesting changes for improvement, using his finely honed editorial skills as the long time editor of *Current Therapy.*

A special thanks to Richard Blum, a master of his craft.

The knowledge, skills, and compassion, of my physicians and their nurses at The University of Iowa--namely Rohan Garje, MD, Rebecca Davis, MD, and Lee Alward, MD—have given me the opportunity to tell the stories of the doctors, my former teachers and friends.

Finally, I thank Steven H. Semken, for his patience and encouragement in writing this narrative. His work with his Ice Cube Press has made available my stories of growing up in affordable housing in Iowa City, *The House of Moffitt*, enjoying adventures boating with friends on the Mississippi River, *Riverin'*, and recording my tribute to my father's contributions to medicine, *Iowa Trailblazer.*

Appendix

The doctors, whose stories tell of their work to improve the care of patients with serious illness:

1. Enrico Fermi, (Scuola Normale '22PhD)
   Herbert Anderson, ('45PhD)
2. Leon O. Jacobson, ('39 MD)††††
   Clarence Lushbaugh, ('48MD)
   Eugene Goldwasser, ('50 PhD)
   Walter Fried, ('58MD)
   Louis F. Plzak, Jr., ('58 MD)
3. Clifford W. Gurney, ('51MD)
   Paul E. Steiner, ('32MD)
   Richard K. Blaisdell, ('48MD)
   John E. Kasik, ('54MD)
4. Sanford B. Krantz, ('59MD)
5. William E. Adams, (UI '26MD)
   Huberta M. (Livingston) Adams, (UI '28MD)
   Peter V. Moulder, Jr., ('45MD)
6. Janet D. Rowley, ('49MD)
7. Henry T. Ricketts, (Harvard '27MD)
   Henry L. Wildberger, ('51MD)
   Randolph W. Seed, ('60 MD)
8. Ernest Beutler, ('50MD)
9. Alf S. Alving, (UM, MD '27)
10. Kenneth M. Brinkhous, (UI, MD '32)
11. Robin D. Powell, ('57MD)
    Allan L. Lorincz, ('47MD)
12. Charles B. Huggins, (Harvard '24MD)
    Cornelius Vermeulen, MD

---

††††('39MD) = indicates the year of the 20th century The University of Chicago awarded the degree, unless otherwise noted

Bibliography

Segre, Gino & Hoerlin, Bettina: *The Pope of Physics, Enrico Fermi and Birth of the Atomic Age*, Henry Holt & Company, New York, 2016, pp. 352.

Wallace, Chris with Mitch Weiss: *Countdown 1945, The Extraordinary Story of the Atomic Bomb and the 116 Days That Changed the World*, Avid Reader Press (An Imprint of Simon & Schuster, Inc.), New York, London, 2020, pp. 312.

Goldwasser, Eugene: *JAKE, Leon O. Jacobson, M.D., The Life and Work of a Distinguished Medical Scientist, Science* History Publications, Sagamore Beach, MA, 2006, pp. 83.

Masterson, Karen M.: *The Malaria Project, The U.S. Government's Secret Mission to Find a Miracle Cure*; New American Library, New York, 2014, pp. 405.

DeGowin, Elmer L., Hardin, Robert C., and Alsever, John B.: *Blood Transfusion*, W.B. Saunders Company, Philadelphia & London, 1949, pp.587.

DeGowin, Richard L.: *Iowa Trailblazer, Contributions to Medicine by Elmer DeGowin*, Ice Cube Press, LLC, North Liberty, IA, 2019, pp. 60.

Steiner, Paul E.: *Medical-Military Portraits of Union and Confederate Generals*, Whitmore Publishing Co, Philadelphia, 1968, pp. 342.

The University of Chicago, Division of Biological Sciences and the Pritzker School of Medicine, 1997 Alumni Directory, Bernard C. Harris Publishing Company, New York, 1997, pp.299.

About the Author

Richard L. DeGowin, MD, FACP, Professor Emeritus, Department of Internal Medicine, Division of Hematology, The University of Iowa, lives in Iowa City, Iowa, where he grew up. He received his MD from The University of Chicago in 1959. During his senior year in medical school, he was elected to the AOA Medical Honor Society. That was the same year his father, Elmer L. DeGowin, MD, MACP, was elected to membership in AOA as a senior faculty member in The University of Iowa College of Medicine, "making it the hard way." After three years' residency/fellowship in Internal Medicine at The University of Chicago, Richard DeGowin accepted a commission as Captain, U.S. Medical Corps, assigned, in 1963, to Walter Reed Army Institute of Research with duty at the University of Chicago-Army Medical Research Project.

At his discharge from two years' active duty in the Army, he was named Assistant Professor of Medicine and Project Supervisor, Argonne Cancer Research Hospital, The University of Chicago. While he served on the faculty for the next three-and-a-half years, he received a Research Career Development Award from the NIH.

He returned to Iowa City as Associate Professor of Medicine, Section of Hematology, with a joint appointment in Radiology and the Radiation Research Laboratory, and as Attending Physician at The University of Iowa Hospitals and Clinics, and at the Veterans Administration Hospital. He is the Founding Director of The University of Iowa Cancer Center.

He served as coauthor with his father for the first four editions of *DeGowin's Diagnostic Examination*. The third edition, published in 1976, was adopted by all American medical schools, half the Canadian schools of medicine, the schools of Osteopathy and Chiropractic,

Physician Assistant Programs, and Nursing Colleges. Now in its tenth edition, published by McGraw-Hill, it has been in print 55 years, with 12 translations into 7 foreign languages: German, French, Italian, Spanish, Portuguese, Greek, and Chinese. McGraw-Hill announced the release of the eleventh edition of *DeGowin's Diagnostic Examination* in December 2020.

Dr. DeGowin received the Laureate Award from the Iowa Chapter of the American College of Physicians. While attending his 50th Year Medical Class Reunion in Chicago, he received the Distinguished Service Award from The University of Chicago. Since his retirement, Ice Cube Press published several of his books: memoirs, *The House of Moffitt*, a story of growing up in Iowa City's affordable housing, and *Riverin'*, a tale of his family's adventures house-boating on the Upper Mississippi River; a tribute to his father, *Iowa Trailblazer, Contributions to Medicine by Elmer DeGowin*; and fiction, *Murder on the Mississippi*.